AF597686

Practical Management of Eye Problems:
GLAUCOMA, STRABISMUS, VISUAL FIELDS

Practical Management of Eye Problems: GLAUCOMA, STRABISMUS, VISUAL FIELDS

FREDERICK HAMPTON ROY, M.D., F.A.C.S.
Department of Ophthalmology,
University of Arkansas Medical Center;
Little Rock Veterans Administration Hospital;
Arkansas Childrens Hospital;
Little Rock, Arkansas

LEA & FEBIGER Philadelphia • 1975

Library of Congress Cataloging in Publication Data

Roy, Frederick Hampton.

Practical management of eye problems: glaucoma, strabismus, visual fields.

Bibliography: p.

1. Eye-Examination. 2. Strabismus. 3. Glaucoma.
I. Title. [DNLM: 1. Glaucoma–Therapy.
2. Strabismus–Therapy. 3. Visual fields. WW290 R88p 1974]
RE75.R68 1974 617.7 74-3283

ISBN 0-8121-0501-X

Published in Great Britain by Henry Kimpton Publishers, London

PRINTED IN THE UNITED STATES OF AMERICA

TO my wife Nancy.

TO all my children.

TO Dr. Fritz Fraunfelder for his assistance through the thick and thin of it.

TO Dr. John Fulmer for his ability to identify applicable patient problems and make practical plans to solve those problems.

TO Dr. Winston Warr for his lucid and interesting presentation of the problem method and penetrating analysis of this material.

TO Dr. Alice Deutsch in memory of an excellent teacher and a superb ophthalmologist.

Preface

This is a plan book of *one* way to handle problems of glaucoma, strabismus, and visual fields. It is *not* of course the *only* way. Each treatment decision should be tempered with clinical judgment.

The information in the strabismus monograph was developed over the last three years and through six revisions. It was the outgrowth of our residents' difficulty in grasping strabismus. We had chosen intelligent, interested residents, so we felt that their ability was not in question. After looking critically at how strabismus was presented, what information was available, and how strabismus cases were treated, we developed the material contained herein. The residents now appear to grasp the problem with greater ease.

Soon after we began our task, we became aware of other efforts in medicine for an organized approach to the medical record. These concepts may be explored further through *Problem Oriented Diagnosis* by Lawrence Weed and *Clinical Judgment* by A. R. Feinstein.

It is envisioned that this text, in its scope, should cover the 85th percentile of common ophthalmic problems of glaucoma, strabismus and visual fields. In its simplicity, it should allow a differential diagnosis, a specific diagnosis, a check on other clinical manifestations, a plan book outlining management for specific problems subject to change by clinical judgment, and a source of reference material for futher reading. As was *Ocular Differential Diagnosis*, it was designed to fit into the problem-oriented method. I would welcome all comments to help improve it for futher editions.

A concept with great validity is "The physician (ophthalmologist) is not an oracle of knowledge, but a guidance system."

The ophthalmologist should not be expected to carry all the knowledge he needs "upstairs." His primary role is to decide how problems should be managed. Our book is used in the examining room during the patient examination to help outline the problems and decide the plans for taking care of them.

Many individuals, including Doctors S. Wilson, J. Sneed, J. Parker, M. Parker, J. Lyford, G. Schroeder, P. Wilson, J. Massey, J. McDonald, J. Landers, and H. Thomas, have aided substantially in the preparation of this text. My thanks are especially due to Dr. Roger Hiatt, Miss Mary Wackerhagen and Mrs. Claire Silvera for their suggestions and encouragement.

This monograph would not have been a reality without the persistent and meticulous secretarial and proofreading efforts of Mrs. Diane Butler, Mrs. Renee Massey, Mrs. Pat Baxter, and Mr. Steve Elrod.

Little Rock, Arkansas

FREDERICK HAMPTON ROY, M.D.

How to Use This Book

This book can be used easily and quickly by following the directions below. Assume you are presented with a glaucoma, strabismus, or visual field problem.

1. If you are unsure how to work up the problem, turn to the data base to determine the amount of data needed to make decisions. With this information, go to either the Diagnostic Decisions or Algorithm, which will help you decide the specific problem. For example, an esotropia problem is presented to you. Consult the
   A. Strabismus data base (p. 99)
   B. Esotropia–Diagnostic Decisions (p. 111) or Eso Algorithm (p. 112) which refers you to
   C. Specific esotropia problem management as A esotropia (p. 132)
2. If you have already decided on the specific problem, such as A esotropia, you may
   A. Turn to the table of contents preceding the section to find the page number on which A esotropia management is discussed, or
   B. Look for A esotropia in the index at the back of the book.

Introduction

Within the last decade there have been a great number of changes in general medicine and in ophthalmology. All physicians have the responsibility to find better ways to gather data, delineate problems and treat these problems.[1] Standardization of medical terminology and computerization of medical records have been additional reasons to explore problem-oriented medical records.[2]

The revolutionary system explained in this introductory chapter has been developed within the last fifteen years by Dr. Lawrence Weed to turn the patient's medical record into a dynamic instrument for structuring medical care. "It raises the medical record to the level of a scientific manuscript and makes it a central tool in medical education and in quality control of medical care. The system, in addition, facilitates computerization of the medical record."[3] This structuring of the medical record has been used extensively in the United States; numerous medical schools have switched over to the system and many separate, private and veterans hospitals are currently using it. The structured problem-oriented medical record is a constructive way to decrease many of the difficulties currently occurring in medicine, as: those medical problems being dealt with out of context, inefficiency in practice, the difference in the quality and quantity of care received by inpatients and outpatients, lack of continuity of care, the apparent neglect of principles of basic science, inefficiency in education, and finally the absence of meaningful audit in the practice of medicine.[4, 5]

Dr. Weed's plan encompasses four phases of medical action: (1) the collection of data (data base), (2) the formulation of a list of all problems, (3) the development of plans and treatment for each problem, and (4) the follow-up through the use of numbered and titled progress notes for each problem.

The *data base* is an initial collection of information about the patient (Table 1). The size and thrust of the data base depend

Table 1. DATA BASE

A. History
   1. Chief complaint
   2. Patient profile
   3. Related social data
   4. Present illness
   5. Past history
   6. System review

B. Physical examination

C. Laboratory reports

to a great extent on the type of specialist and the interest of the individual collecting the data. It is important that the data base be specified precisely, so that one can look at the medical record and know which questions were asked and which were not, which parts of the physical examination were performed and which were not. This assures some degree of quality control in medical practice, and each physician therefore is not left to create his own standards. The data base should consist of six basic elements: (1) chief complaint, (2) patient profile, (3) present illnesses, (4) past history and systems review, (5) physical examination, and (6) reports of laboratory work.

On the basis of the ocular data base a *problem list* can then be constructed (Table 2). The physician can list all of the patient's problems, past as well as present, social and psychiatric as well as medical. The problem list to a large extent will depend on the field of interest of the individual drawing it up and on the level of his understanding.

Four types of problems should be noted on the problem list: (1) medical, (2) social, (3) demographic, and (4) psychiatric. Medical problems can be such things as a diagnosis (exophthalmos),

Table 2. PROBLEM NUMBERED AND TITLED. FORMULATION OF ALL PROBLEMS, ACTIVE AND INACTIVE

A. Medical problems
   1. Diagnosis—as strabismus
   2. Physiological findings—as esotropia, greater at near than distance
   3. Symptom—as closing one eye outside in the sunlight
   4. Physical finding—as retina dragged temporally
   5. Abnormal laboratory finding—as elevated sedimentation rate

B. Social problems—as bankruptcy

C. Demographic problems (health problems)—as environmental pollution

D. Psychiatric problems (in nontechnical language)—as nervousness

a physiological finding (cloudy cornea), a symptom or physical finding (photophobia or ciliary flush), or an abnormal laboratory finding (elevated sedimentation rate). Social problems might include such things as bankruptcy or delinquency. Demographic problems might include health hazards (industrial pollution). Psychiatric problems should be described in nontechnical language.

After a problem list has been formulated, a differential diagnosis list can be consulted to determine the entities exhibiting these symptoms or signs. The recently published book *Ocular Differential Diagnosis* was designed to fit into the problem-oriented method.[6]

Plans for the management of each problem, keyed by number to the problem list, should then be formulated.[7, 8, 9] Plans can fall into three categories: (1) plans for collecting further data in order to establish a diagnosis or facilitate management, (2) plans for treatment with specific procedures or drugs, (3) plans for education of the patient about his illness or his part in managing it.

The progress notes should be written in a form which relates unmistakably to the problem. Each note should be preceded by the number and title of the appropriate problem. This method immediately tells the reader that it is the progress of the subject under discussion. Each problem-oriented section of the progress notes consists of any or all of the following elements: (1) subjective data, (2) objective data, (3) assessment, (4) plan. This has been shortened to SOAP–S(ubjective), O(bjective), A(ssessment), and P(lan).

Subjective data include the symptomatic information from the patient. Objective data include valuable physical findings and laboratory work which support the problem. The creation of a flow sheet might be meaningful to follow the objective data. The interpretation or assessment is made from that section of the progress notes. The doctor should state his thinking, any disagreements which have arisen, and, if applicable, the opinions of other expert consultants regarding the issue. Immediate plans, the plans section of the progress notes, should state any modifications or additions that have been made to the initial plans.

Nurses' notes, social service notes, physical medicine notes, residents' notes, operative notes, consultants' notes can be put in this same type of format to assist in solving the problem at hand. The discharge summary should also be problem oriented. Only the history and physical and laboratory information necessary in the future analysis or management of a problem should be included.

1. Parrott, M. H.: The American Physician's Responsibility. Trans. Amer. Acad. Ophthal. Otolaryng. 75:1139-1144, 1971.
2. Savett, L. A.: A Computer-Compatible Solution to the Medical Record Problem. Trans. Amer. Acad. Ophthal. Otolaryng. 75:1120-1125, 1971.
3. Weed, L. L.: Medical Records, Medical Education and Patient Care. Chicago, Press of Case Western University, Year Book Medical Publishers, 1971.
4. Weed, L. L.: Medical Records that Guide and Teach. Part I. New Eng. J. Med. 278:593-599, 1968. Part II. New Eng. J. Med. 278:652-657, 1968.
5. Hurst, J. W.: Ten Reasons Why Lawrence Weed is Right. New Eng. J. Med. 284:51, 1971.
6. Roy, F. H.: Ocular Differential Diagnosis, 2nd ed. Philadelphia, Lea & Febiger, 1975.
7. Arsham, G. M. and Spivey, B. E.: An Integrated System of Health Care and Medical Education. *In:* Blodi, F. C.: Current Concepts in Ophthalmology, Vol. III. St. Louis, C. V. Mosby, 1972, pp. 214-220.
8. Colenbrander, A.: Information Systems in Ophthalmology. *In:* Blodi, F. C.: Current Concepts in Ophthalmology, Vol. III. St. Louis, C. V. Mosby, 1972, pp. 221-231.
9. Hurst, J. W. and Walker, H. K.: The Problem-Oriented System. New York, Medcom Inc., 1972.

Glaucoma Problems

Glaucoma Problems

CONTENTS

Glaucoma Problems

PRESENTING INFANTILE GLAUCOMA PROBLEMS

1. Tearing (epiphora)
2. Photophobia
3. Blepharospasm
4. Corneal enlargement
5. Corneal haziness
6. Elevated intraocular pressure (constant or transitory)
7. Optic disc changes

INFANTILE GLAUCOMA SUSPECT

1. Epiphora
2. Photophobia
3. Blepharospasm
4. Corneal edema
5. Corneal enlargement
6. Tears in Descemet's membrane
7. Deep anterior chamber
8. Optic disc changes of glaucoma
9. Iridodonesis and subluxation of lens
10. Strabismus secondary to decreased vision
11. Aniridia or posterior embryotoxon

Kolker, A. E. and Hetherington, J.: Becker-Shaffer's Diagnosis and Therapy of the Glaucomas. St. Louis, C. V. Mosby, 1970, pp. 259-263.

CONDITIONS SIMULATING CONGENITAL GLAUCOMA

1. Inflammation
   A. Syphilitic interstitial keratitis
   B. Intrauterine gonorrhea keratitis
   C. Smallpox and chickenpox viruses–intrauterine
   D. Fetal iritis or uveitis
   E. Blepharitis, keratoconjunctivitis, and keratitis on a chemical, allergic, bacterial, or viral basis
2. Metabolic disorders
   A. Familial lipoidosis
   B. Cystinosis or cystine storage disease
   C. Hurler's disease (MPSI), Morquio Brailsford disease (MPSIV), Scheie's disease (MPSV), and Maroteaux Lamy syndrome (MPSVI)
   D. Porphyria
3. Congenital idiopathic corneal edema
4. Blue sclerotic syndrome
5. Riley-Day syndrome
6. Megalocornea
7. Myopia
8. Anterior corneal staphyloma
9. Cornea plana
10. Keratoconus
11. Keratoectasia
12. Intraocular tumor such as retinoblastoma or diktyoma
13. Bloch-Sulzberger syndrome (incontinentia pigmenti)
14. Congenital corneal dystrophy
15. Birth injury such as breaks in Descemet's membrane
16. Trisomy 13-15 syndrome
17. Corneal amyloidosis
18. Corneal xanthomas
19. von Gierke's disease (glycogen disease)
20. Congenital anomalies as sclerocornea

Becker, B. and Shaffer, R. N.: Diagnosis and Therapy of Glaucoma. St. Louis, C. V. Mosby, 1970, pp. 263-264.

Geeraets, W. J.: Ocular Syndromes, 2nd ed. Philadelphia, Lea & Febiger, 1969, pp. 221-222.

Howard, R. O. and Abrahams, I. W.: Sclerocornea. Amer. J. Ophthal. 71:1254-1260, 1971.

Kenyon, K. R., et al.: The Systemic Mucopolysaccharidoses. Amer. J. Ophthal. 73:811-833, 1972.

Kwitko, M. L.: Glaucoma in Infants and Children. Mod. Med. Canad. 23:1-8, 1968.

Liebman, S. D., Crocker, A. C., and Geiser, C. F.: Corneal Xanthomas in Childhood. Arch. Ophthal. 76:220-221, 1966.

McPherson, S. D., Jr., Kiffney, G. T., and Freed, C. C.: Corneal Amyloidosis. Amer. J. Ophthal. 62:1025, 1966.

Rodger, F. C. and Sinclair, H. M.: Metabolic and Nutritional Eye Diseases. Springfield, Charles C Thomas, 1969, p. 104.

Townsend, W. M.: Congenital Corneal Leukomas. Amer. J. Ophthal. 77:80-86, 1974.

PRESENTING ADULT GLAUCOMA PROBLEMS

1. Asymptomatic with an elevated intraocular pressure
2. Family history of glaucoma
3. Suspicious history
   - A. Previous glaucoma therapy
   - B. Foggy vision
   - C. Colored halos around lights
   - D. Asthenopia
   - E. Pain and redness of eye
   - F. Transient blackout of vision—few minutes to an hour

ADULT GLAUCOMA SUSPECT

1. Applanation reading 21 mm Hg or higher
2. Schiotz scale reading 4.0/5.5 or 6.25/7.5 gm weight
3. Visual field changes suggestive of glaucoma
4. Asymmetry of optic disc or cup/disc ratio over 0:4
5. Family history of glaucoma

6. Intraocular pressure elevation following use of topical corticosteroids
7. High myopia
8. Thyrotropic exophthalmos
9. Retinal vein occlusion
10. Retinal detachment
11. Krukenberg's spindle and/or dense trabecular pigment band
12. Endothelial dystrophy of cornea
13. Pseudoexfoliation of lens capsule
14. Diabetes mellitus
15. Shallow anterior chamber (slit to Grade 1)
16. Severe injury to one eye which might give recessed angle with glaucoma

Kolker, A. E. and Hetherington, J.: Becker-Shaffer's Diagnosis and Therapy of the Glaucomas. St. Louis, C. V. Mosby, 1970, pp. 207-210.

GLAUCOMA DATA BASE—infantile and adult

1. History
   - A. Family history of glaucoma
   - B. Pregnancy, labor and delivery and birth weight (infantile only)
   - C. Early and current development (infantile only)
   - D. General health (operations, hospitalizations, current medications, allergies)
   - E. Systemic diseases including diabetes mellitus, vascular disease, hypertension, thyroid disease, anemia, hypotensive episodes, arrhythmias
   - F. Time of onset of presenting problem
   - G. Course (intermittent or constant, progression)
2. Examination
   - A. Visual acuity (with and without correction, both distance and near)
     - (1) Fixation pattern—central or eccentric, maintained or not maintained. If thought to be eccentric, visuoscope

determines position as paramacular or parafoveal (infantile only)

(2) Linear Snellen

(3) Isolated E

B. Binocular alignment—extraocular movement (cardinal fields of gaze, cover-uncover and cover-cover test)

C. Inspection and biomicroscopy

(1) Lids

(2) Conjunctiva

(3) Cornea—especially horizontal corneal diameter and applanation tonometry

(4) Anterior chamber—clarity and depth

(5) Pupil

(6) Lens

(7) Vitreous cavity

D. Tonometry (see p. 23)—an intraocular pressure over 22 mm Hg should be looked at critically. Test before gonioscopy

E. Gonioscopy (see p. 29)

(1) Angle width and iris contour

(2) Pigmentation of trabecular meshwork

(3) Presence of blood in Schlemm's canal, peripheral anterior synechiae, and neovascularization of chamber angle

F. Fundus examination

(1) Vessels

(2) Macula

(3) Background pigmentation

(4) Optic disc evaluation (see p. 24)

a. Size disc and cup

b. Shape disc and cup

c. Cup/disc ratio

d. Vessels on disc

G. Manifest or cycloplegic refraction

H. Visual field (see p. 28). Tangent screen most frequently used for glaucoma evaluation

I. Tonography—may be of value (see p. 38)

UNILATERAL GLAUCOMA

1. Trauma
   - A. Contusion
     - (1) Angle deformity or recession (see p.71)
     - (2) Hemolytic glaucoma (see p. 73)
     - (3) Scarring, vascularization, and peripheral anterior synechiae of the anterior chamber
     - (4) Iritis and trabeculitis (see p.88)
     - (5) Phacolytic glaucoma (see p. 90)
   - B. Perforating wound
     - (1) Peripheral anterior synechiae and scarring of the anterior chamber (see p. 75)
     - (2) Phacolytic glaucoma (see p. 90)
   - C. Intraocular foreign body
     - (1) Siderosis bulbi, chalcosis and other heavy-metal implantation
     - (2) Chronic inflammation
   - D. Chemical burn
     - (1) Keratouveitis
     - (2) Phacolytic glaucoma (see p. 90)
2. Intraocular tumor with secondary glaucoma–benign cysts of iris, ciliary processes, malignant melanoma, pigment from tumor or cyst closing off trabecular meshwork (see p. 79)
3. Neovascularization of iris and chamber angle (see p. 85)
4. Inflammation
   - A. Anterior uveitis (see p. 88)
     - (1) With peripheral anterior synechiae
     - (2) With open angle including glaucomatocyclitic crisis and heterochromic iridocyclitis
   - B. Corneal
     - (1) Chronic interstitial keratitis
     - (2) Chemical keratitis
     - (3) Chronic keratitis secondary to herpes zoster or herpes simplex (see p. 88)
     - (4) Acute bacterial ulcer of cornea
5. Lens changes
   - A. Phacolytic reaction (see p. 90)

   B. Intumescent lens
   C. Dislocated lens (p. 92)
   D. Associated with pseudoexfoliation of anterior lens capsule (see p. 68)

6. Early-onset uniocular open-angle glaucoma (see p. 60)
7. Association with extradural hemorrhage, intracranial aneurysm or fistula
8. Carotid-cavernous sinus fistula or other entities with extraocular venous congestion (see p. 72)
9. Acute angle-closure glaucoma—other eye may be predisposed to same event (see p. 75)
10. Corticoste oid glaucoma—(see p. 70)
11. Essential atrophy of the iris with glaucoma—atrophy of the iris, distortion of the pupil, iridocorneal synechiae, and unilateral corneal edema (see p. 83)
12. Retinal detachment
13. Ophthalmic vein thrombosis
14. Cavernous sinus thrombosis

Boniuk, M.: The Ocular Manifestations of Ophthalmic Vein and Aseptic Cavernous Sinus Thrombosis. Trans. Amer. Acad. Ophthal. Otolaryng. 76:1519-1534, 1972.

Chandler, P. A. and Grant, W. M.: Lectures on Glaucoma. Philadelphia, Lea & Febiger, 1965, pp. 291-295.

de Roetth, A., Jr.: Glaucomatocyclitic Crisis. Amer. J. Ophthal. 69: 370-371, 1970.

Drance, S. M., Wheeley, C., and Pattullo, M.: Uniocular Open-Angle Glaucoma. Amer. J. Ophthal. 65:891, 1968.

Koeppen, A. H., Madonick, M. J., and Barest, M. D.: Acute Unilateral Glaucoma Associated with Extradural Hemorrhage. Amer. J. Ophthal. 63:1696, 1967.

Miles, D. R. and Boniuk, M.: Pathogenesis of Unilateral Glaucoma. Amer. J. Ophthal. 62:493, 1966.

Roy, F. H.: Ocular Differential Diagnosis, 2nd ed. Philadelphia, Lea & Febiger, 1975, pp. 273-274.

GLAUCOMA DUE TO INTRAOCULAR INFLAMMATION

1. Acute uveitis (see p. 88)
2. Herpetic keratitis and uveitis (see p. 88)
3. Anterior ond posterior uveitis (see p. 88)
   A. Toxoplasmosis
   B. Peripheral uveitis (cyclitis)
   C. Syphilis
   D. Tuberculosis
   E. Sarcoidosis
   F. Vogt-Koyanagi-Harada syndrome
   G. Unknown
4. Recurrent and chronic iridocyclitis (see p. 88)
   A. Glaucomatocyclic crisis
   B. Heterochromic iridocyclitis
   C. Sarcoid uveitis
   D. Pars planitis
5. Phacolytic glaucoma (see p. 90)
   A. Hypermature cataract
   B. Immature cataract
   C. Completely dislocated hypermature cataract and glaucoma
   D. Phacolytic glaucoma due to retained lens cortex

Chandler, P. A. and Grant, W. M.: Lectures on Glaucoma. Philadelphia, Lea & Febiger, 1965, pp. 244-267.

Schlaegel, T. F.: Essentials of Uveitis. Boston, Little, Brown & Co., 1969, p. 2.

"APHAKIC" GLAUCOMA (glaucoma in aphakia)

1. Primary open-angle glaucoma (see p. 60)
2. Associated with pseudoexfoliation in aphakia (see p. 68)
3. Peripheral anterior synechiae from loss of vitreous, prolapse of iris, incarceration of iris or lens capsule in wound or absent anterior chamber (see p. 80)

4. Pupillary block
5. Vitreous filling the anterior chamber
6. Immediate postoperative reaction after intracapsular extraction from traumatic iritis causing a trabeculitis
7. Epithelialization of the anterior chamber
8. Prolonged postoperative inflammation in aphakia in both intracapsular and extracapsular extraction (see p. 90)
9. Alpha chymotrypsin-induced glaucoma from zonule fragment impeding aqueous outflow

Chandler, D. A. and Grant, W. M.: Lectures on Glaucoma. Philadelphia, Lea & Febiger, 1965, pp. 234-243.

Kolker, A. and Hetherington, J.: Becker-Shaffer's Diagnosis and Therapy of the Glaucomas, 3rd ed. St. Louis, C. V. Mosby, 1970, pp. 225-243.

CORNEAL OPACIFICATION IN INFANCY—differential diagnosis

1. Congenital glaucoma (see p. 47)
2. Inflammation
   - A. Syphilitic interstitial keratitis
   - B. Intrauterine gonorrhea keratitis
   - C. Smallpox and chickenpox viruses–intrauterine
   - D. Fetal iritis or uveitis
   - E. Blepharitis, keratoconjunctivitis, and keratitis on a chemical, allergic, bacterial, or viral basis
   - F. Rubella syndrome
   - G. Herpes simplex
   - H. Riley-Day syndrome
3. Metabolic errors
   - A. Mucopolysaccharidoses
     - (1) Hurler's (type I)
     - (2) Morquio-Brailsford (type IV)
     - (3) Scheie's (type V)
     - (4) Maroteaux-Lamy (type VI)

B. Lowe's syndrome
C. Corneal lipoidosis—later
D. Cystinosis—later
E. Corneal amyloidosis
F. Corneal xanthomas
G. Von Gierke's disease
H. Mucolipidosis
(1) Generalized gangliosidosis (GM_1-gangliosidosis I and II)
(2) MLS I (lipomucopolysaccharidosis)
(3) MLS III (pseudoHurler polydystrophy)

4. Congenital malformations
A. Anterior chamber cleavage syndromes
(1) Congenital central anterior synechiae
(2) Rieger's syndrome
(3) Axenfeld's syndrome
(4) Peters' anomaly
(5) Congenital anterior staphyloma
B. Sclerocornea
C. Dermoid tumors

5. Chromosomal aberrations
A. Mongolism (Down's syndrome)—trisomy 21
B. Trisomy 13-15 (Patau's syndrome)

6. Birth trauma including rupture of Descemet membrane

7. Corneal dystrophy as congenital hereditary corneal dystrophy

Ching, F. C.: Corneal Opacification in Infancy. Med. Coll. Va. Quart. 8:230-240, 1972.

Emery, J. M., et al.: GM1-Gangliosidosis: Ocular and Pathological Manifestations. Arch. Ophthal. 85:1677-1787, 1971.

Fergin, R. D. and Caplan, D. B.: Corneal Opacities in Infancy and Childhood. J. Pediat. 69:383-392, 1966.

Geeraets, W. J.: Ocular Syndromes. Philadelphia, Lea & Febiger, 1969, pp. 221-222.

Goldberg, M. F., Scott, C. I., and McKusick, V. A.: Hydrocephalus and Papilledema in the Maroteaux-Lamy Syndrome (Mucopolysaccharidosis Type VI). Amer. J. Ophthal. 69:969-974, 1970.

Grayson, M. and Keates, R. H.: Manual of Diseases of the Cornea. Boston, Little, Brown & Co., 1969, p. 295.

Harboyan, G., et al.: Congenital Corneal Dystrophy. Arch. Ophthal. 85:27-32, 1971.

Howard, R. O., and Abrahms, I. W.: Sclerocornea. Amer. J. Ophthal. 71:1254-1260, 1971.

Kenyon, K. R. and Sensenbrenner, J. A.: Mucolipidosis II (I-Cell Disease): Ultrastructure Observations of Conjunctiva and Skin. Invest. Ophthal. 10:555-567, 1971.

Kolker, A. E. and Hetherington, J.: Becker-Shaffer's Diagnosis and Therapy of the Glaucomas, 3rd ed. St. Louis, C. V. Mosby, 1970.

Liebman, S. D., Crocker, A. C., and Geiser, C. F.: Corneal Xanthomas in Childhood. Arch. Ophthal. 76:221-229, 1966.

McPherson, S. D., Jr., Kiffney, G. T., and Freed, C. C.: Corneal Amyloidosis. Amer. J. Ophthal. 62:1025, 1966.

Reese, A. B. and Ellsworth, R.: The Anterior Chamber Cleavage Syndrome. Arch. Ophthal. 75:307, 1966.

Roy, F. H.: Ocular Differential Diagnosis, 2nd ed. Philadelphia, Lea & Febiger, 1975, pp. 264-266.

CONGENITAL GLAUCOMA ASSOCIATED WITH OCULAR AND SYSTEMIC ANOMALIES

1. Ocular anomalies
   - A. Iridocorneal dysgenesis (anterior chamber cleavage syndrome)
     - (1) Posterior embryotoxon of Axenfeld—anterior displacement of Schwalbe's line, iris strand attaching to prominent Schwalbe's line, hypertelorism and skeletal abnormalities
     - (2) Rieger's syndrome—hypoplasia of the anterior stromal leaf of the iris, iridotrabecular adhesions, and posterior embryotoxon
     - (3) Dense central corneal opacity with iris synechiae
   - B. Essential iris atrophy—localized area (or areas) of atrophy beginning in the stroma and eventually involving all layers (see p. 83)
   - C. Aniridia—absence of the iris, never complete; gonioscopy shows a rudimentary iris (see p. 50)
   - D. Pigmentary glaucoma—idiopathic atrophy of the pigment

epithelium of the iris, which is deposited on the lens capsule at the insertion of the zonular fibers, the anterior surface of the iris, the corneal endothelium in the form of Krukenberg's spindle, and in the angle, especially in the trabecular meshwork (see p. 69)

E. Megalocornea—hereditary enlargement of cornea

F. Microcornea—in the hyperopic eyes the anterior chamber is often shallow and the angles narrow; an acute attack of glaucoma is possible (see p. 75)

G. Microphthalmos—autosomal dominant and recessive inheritance trait

H. Spherophakia (microphakia)—lens is small and spherical in shape, and its edges can be identified through the dilated pupil; a high degree of myopia may be present

I. Myopia

J. Retinitis pigmentosa

K. Coloboma of the iris

L. Polycoria

M. Sclerocornea

N. Hemangioma of the choroid (see p. 52)

O. Retinoblastoma

P. Retrolental fibroplasia

Q. Persistent hyperplastic primary vitreous

R. Anterior uveitis (see p. 88)

S. Heterochromic iridocyclitis

T. Trauma

U. Congenital cataract

2. Systemic anomalies

A. Phakomatoses—disseminated hamartomas that have eye, skin, and brain involvement in common

(1) Neurofibromatosis (von Recklinghausen's disease)—neurofibromas in various parts of the body, skin pigmentation (cafe-au-lait spots), and skeletal changes such as pseudarthrosis. Ocular findings may include ptosis and neurofibroma of the skin of the eyelids and also of the uvea

(2) Encephalotrigeminal angiomatosis of Sturge-Weber—intracranial angioma associated with facial and

choroidal angiomas, which are homolateral and present at birth (see p. 52)

(3) Tuberous sclerosis—adenoma sebaceum

(4) von Hippel-Lindau disease (angiomatosis retinae)

B. Heritable disorders of connective tissue

(1) Marfan's syndrome—long, thin extremities, diffuse dilatation, and at times dissection of aorta and/or ectopia lentis

(2) Weil-Marchesani syndrome – brachymorphism and shortness of stature, with round head, pug nose, depressed nasal bridge, and short, pudgy hands and fingers; ectopia lentis

(3) Homocystinuria arterial disease, arachnodactylia, ectopia lentis, mental retardation, venous thrombosis, and pulmonary embolism

(4) Hurler's disease (MPS I)—corneal opacities, true megalocornea, congenital glaucoma, pigmentary retinopathy

(5) Rendu-Osler-Weber disease (telangiectasia of skin)

C. Lowe's syndrome (oculocerebrorenal syndrome)—systemic acidosis, organic aciduria, decreased ability to produce ammonia in the kidneys, renal rickets, generalized hypotonicity, retardation, glaucoma, and cataracts

D. Pierre Robin syndrome—hypoplasia of the mandible, glossoptosis, cleft palate, high myopia, retinal detachment, glaucoma, cataracts, and microphthalmia

E. Hallerman-Streiff syndrome—dyscephaly, birdlike facies, localized hypotrichosis, localized atrophy of the skin, and bilateral microphthalmia with associated severe congenital glaucoma or cataracts

F. Chromosomal disorders

(1) Turner's syndrome—infantilism, webbing of the skin of the neck, equinovarus, dwarfism, and amenorrhea

(2) Trisomy 16-18—failure to thrive, low-set ears, malformed pinnae, mental retardation, hypotonicity, small mouth and mandible, ventricular septal defects, flexion deformities of fingers, partial syndactylia of toes, renal anomalies, congenital glaucoma, optic

atrophy, lenticular opacities, corneal opacities, and ptosis

(3) Trisomy 13-15—malformations of the brain, heart, and viscera; polydactylia, harelip, cleft palate, microphthalmia, retinal dysplasia, iris and ciliary body colobomas, and persistent hyperplastic primary vitreous

(4) Down's syndrome (mongolism) (trisomy 21)

G. Oculodentodigital syndrome (hereditary oculodento-osseous dysplasia)—anomalies of the extremities, mental defects, microphthalmia, coloboma, and glaucoma

H. Pyrophalangeal dyscrasia (Ullrich's syndrome)—cranial deformities, broad nose, small mandible, associated skeletal and visceral abnormalities, bilateral anophthalmia; defects such as microphthalmia, chorioretinal coloboma, complete aniridia, ciliary body hypoplasia, and gross mesodermal abnormalities of the anterior chamber

I. Congenital melanosis oculi—unilateral hyperpigmentation of the uveal tract, sclera, and, occasionally, of the periorbital skin (nevus of Ota)

J. Juvenile xanthogranuloma—widespread yellow to orange skin nodules that occur shortly after birth; occasionally these lesions occur in the iris and ciliary body and are prone to cause anterior chamber hemorrhage, giving rise to secondary glaucoma

K. Idiopathic infantile hypoglycemia—neonatal hypoglycemia, nasolacrimal duct obstruction, congenital cataracts, squint, cortical blindness, atrophy of the optic disc, congenital glaucoma

L. Congenital rubella syndrome

M. Syphilis

N. Toxoplasmosis

Kwitko, M. L.: Glaucoma in Infants and Children. Mod. Med. Canad. 23:1-8, 1968.

Scheie, H.: Surgical and Medical Management of Congenital Anomalies of the Eye. New Orleans Academy of Ophthalmology. St. Louis, C. V. Mosby, 1966, pp. 356-360.

Roy, F. H.: Ocular Differential Diagnosis, 2nd ed. Philadelphia, Lea & Febiger, 1975, pp. 266-269.

PUPILLARY BLOCK GLAUCOMA

1. Phakic eyes
   - A. Iridolenticular pupillary block (iris bombé) (see p. 91)
   - B. Iridiolenticular block (relative pupillary block) (see p. 75)
   - C. Ciliary block (malignant glaucoma) (see p. 81)
     - (1) Ciliovitreolenticular block
     - (2) Ciliolenticular block
2. Aphakic eyes (see p. 80)
   - A. Aphakic iridovitreal block
     - (1) With a normal hyaloid face
     - (2) With a weak hyaloid membrane
   - B. Ciliovitreal block (continuing malignant glaucoma)

Grant, W. M.: Discussion: Ciliary Block (Malignant) Glaucoma. Trans. Amer. Acad. Ophthal. Otolaryng. 76:60, 1972.

Levene, R.: A New Concept of Malignant Glaucoma. Arch. Ophthal. 87:497, 1972.

Shaffer, R. N.: A Suggested Anatomic Classification to Define the Pupillary Block Glaucoma. Invest. Ophthal. 12:540-542, 1973.

Weiss, D. I. and Shaffer, R. N.: Ciliary Block (Malignant) Glaucoma. Trans. Amer. Acad. Ophthal. Otolaryng. 76:450, 1972.

GLAUCOMA TESTS AND INTERPRETATION

Measurement of Intraocular Pressure

1. Technique
   - A. Schiotz tonometer—With the patient supine, a topical anesthetic is placed on the eye. The lids are carefully held apart and the footplate of the tonometer is centered on the anterior surface of the cornea. The amount of indentation of the tonometer on the cornea is measured in scale units. These units can be converted to millimeters of mercury by the use of a conversion table.
   - B. Applanation tonometer—The patient sits erect in front of the slit lamp following the installation of topical anesthetic and fluorescein. The applanation tonometer is placed on the front surface of the eye. The end-point for measure-

ment is the touching of the inner edge of two semicircles. The intraocular pressure in mm Hg is read directly from the instrument.

C. Horizontal applanation tonometer (Perkins or Draeger)—The principle and technique of the applanation tonometer are the same as those above, except that the individual may be in almost any position.

D. MacKay-Marg electronic tonometer—This is an applanation type of tonometer. Readings are automatically recorded and a permanent record is obtained. The most accurate results are obtained if a topical anesthetic is used.

2. Interpretation

Intraocular pressures over 21 mm Hg applanation and 23 mm Hg Schiotz must be regarded with great suspicion for glaucoma.

3. Elevated intraocular pressure with normal optic disc—differential diagnosis

   A. Systemic hypertension
   B. Excessive water intake
   C. Hyperthyroid
   D. Normal variation
   E. Marked emotional stress
   F. Mechanical factors in checking intraocular pressure
   G. High scleral rigidity
   H. Preglaucoma
   I. Steroid intake (local, systemic)
   J. Ocular hypertension (see p. 60)

Kolker, A. E. and Hetherington, J.: Becker-Shaffer's Diagnosis and Therapy of the Glaucomas. St. Louis, C. V. Mosby, 1970, pp. 55-64.

Phelps, C. D., et al.: Diurnal Variation in Intraocular Pressure. Amer. J. Ophthal. 77:367-377, 1974.

Optic Disc Evaluation

1. Technique

   A. Direct ophthalmoscope—simple, quick, magnified 15X, monocular
   B. Binocular direct ophthalmoscope—binocular, magnified

C. Use of the slit lamp with a Rhuby lens or a fundus contact lens—binocular, magnified, more complex method

D. Indirect ophthalmoscope (especially valuable in high myopia or when the medium is hazy)—minified view, binocular, inverted image

E. Smooth-dome Koeppe contact lens with + 12.00 lens in ophthalmoscope

2. Interpretation—A change may be noted if a photograph, drawing or definite cup/disc ratio observation has been made in the past. Optic disc appearance should correspond to the visual field defect.

A. Size—The cup/disc ratio should be measured either by a drawing or by a decimal system. A cup/disc ratio greater than 0.4 must be looked at very critically to see if a glaucoma problem is present. The horizontal diameter of the physiological cup is compared to the horizontal diameter of the disc. For example, if the cup diameter is 30% of the disc, then the cup/disc ratio is 0.3.

B. Shape—If the shape of the physiological cup is horizontal, this is probably normal. If the cup is vertically oval (the cup extends upward and downward toward the upper and lower poles of the disc, so that the rim of disc tissue is nearest at this location and the cup itself is vertically oval in shape) it is probably abnormal even with a normal pressure. The shape must be compared to that of the other disc.

C. Rim of the optic disc—If the physiological cup extends toward the rim of the optic disc or is eccentrically placed, this should be looked at very critically.

D. Vessel location with the emergence of the vessels not centrally placed—If there is a deviation toward the rim of the cup, or if a vessel loops down out of sight under an overhang, this may be significant. Either is a late change of glaucoma.

E. Color—Pallor is a late change of glaucoma (maximum color contrast and lack of small vessels). The temporal rim is usually the first area to show color change. In general, hyperopic discs show more redness than myopic discs.

F. Assymmetry between the two optic discs is fairly common early in glaucoma. Changes greater than 0.2 cup/disc ratio are rare in normal individuals, except those with congenital anomalies such as hypoplastic nerve or anisometropia.

G. Peripapillary halos represent interference with the posterior ciliary circulation of the disc and peripapillary choroid and may occur with advanced cupping with glaucoma. Many normal people have some degree of peripapillary atrophy or congenital crescents and rings which may be difficult to distinguish.

Armaly, M. F.: Genetic Determinations of Cup/Disc Ratio of the Optic Nerve. Arch. Ophthal. 78:35-43, 1967.

Armaly, M. F. and Sayegh, R. E.: The Cup/Disc Ratio: The Findings of Tonometry and Tonography in the Normal Eye. Arch. Ophthal. 82:191-196, 1969.

Fishman, R. S.: Optic Disc Asymmetry: A Sign of Ocular Hypertension. Arch. Ophthal. 84:590-594, 1970.

Kirsch, R. E. and Anderson, D. R.: Identification of the Glaucomatous Disc. Trans. Amer. Acad. Ophthal. Otolaryng. 77:143-156, 1973.

Kirsch, R. E. and Anderson, D. R.: Clinical Recognition of Glaucomatous Cupping. Amer. J. Ophthal. 75:442-454, 1973.

Read, R. M. and Spaeth, G. L.: The Practical Clinical Appraisal of the Optic Disc in Glaucoma. Trans. Amer. Acad. Ophthal. Otolaryng. 78:255-274, 1974.

Richardson, K. T.: Optic Cup Symmetry in Normal Newborn Infants. Invest. Ophthal. 7:137-140, 1968.

Schwartz, B., Reinstein, N. M., and Lieberman, D. M.: Pallor of the Optic Disc: Quantitative Photographic Evaluation. Arch. Ophthal. 89:278-286, 1973.

Schwartz, B.: Cupping and Pallor of the Optic Disc. Arch. Ophthal. 89:269-274, 1973.

Weisman, R. L., Asseff, C. F., Phelps, C. D., Podos, S. M., and Becker, B.: Vertical Elongation of the Optic Cup in Glaucoma. Trans. Amer. Acad. Ophthal. Otolaryng. 77:157-161, 1973.

3. Glaucomatous atrophy of the optic disc with normal intraocular pressure—cupping of the nerve head with or without optic atrophy and field defects simulating true glaucoma, but without ocular hypertension

A. Primary open-angle glaucoma with large diurnal variation and elevation of intraocular pressure above 22 mm Hg at some time of the day or night (see p. 60)

B. Open-angle glaucoma with low scleral rigidity (following intraocular surgery, associated with myopia and patients receiving miotic therapy) with low-pressure reading with Schiotz tonometry and elevated Goldmann applanation intraocular pressures (see p. 60)
   (1) Myopia
   (2) Thyrotropic exophthalmos
   (3) After ocular surgery
   (4) Use of strong miotics as Phospholine iodide
   (5) Water drinking

C. Previous damage to optic nerve with normal intraocular pressure now, as with prior corticosteroid glaucoma, secondary glaucoma, spontaneously "cured" open-angle glaucoma, or intermittent angle-closure glaucoma. Anterior or posterior synechiae, and pigmented old inflammatory deposits.

D. True low-tension glaucoma (see p. 65)

E. Congenital anomalies of the optic disc
   (1) Oblique insertion of the optic nerve
   (2) Branching of vessels behind the lamina, so that the individual branches appear at the disc margins
   (3) Congenital coloboma of the disc
   (4) Coloboma within the nerve sheath
   (5) Traction of the disc with bowing of the scleral crescent, usually symmetrical

F. Sclerosis or calcification of the internal carotid arteries with pressure on optic nerves or arteriosclerosis of the nutrient vessels of the optic nerve

G. Tumors arising near the chiasm (rare)

H. Syphilitic optic atrophy

I. Open-angle glaucoma with hyposecretion of aqueous humor and decreased facility of outflow. Diagnosed by tonography (see p. 60)

J. "Weak" optic disc which atrophies at normal pressures, or reduced nutrition to optic nerve, as severe blood loss, gastrointestinal bleeding, acute hypotension, myocardial infarction, carotid insufficiency, or pernicious anemia

K. Schnabel's cavernous atrophy

L. Digitalis therapy

Deutsch, A. R.: Differential Characteristics of Low Tension Glaucoma. J. Tenn. Med. Assoc. 54:84-89, 1961.

Drance, S. M., et al.: Studies of Factors Involved in the Production of Low Tension Glaucoma. Arch. Ophthal. 89:457-465, 1973.

Hiatt, R. L., Deutsch, A. R., and Ringer, C.: Low Tension Glaucoma. Ann. Ophthal. 3:85-92, 1971.

Kolker, A. E. and Hetherington, J.: Becker-Shaffer's Diagnosis and Therapy of the Glaucomas, 3rd ed. St. Louis, C. V. Mosby, 1970, pp. 223-225.

McDonald, T. J.: Problems of Low Tension Glaucoma. Trans. Ophthal. Soc. U. K. 87:873-892, 1967.

Vaughan, D., Asbury, T., and Cook, R.: General Ophthalmology, 6th ed. Los Altos, Lange Medical Publishers, 1971, p. 200.

Glaucoma Visual Field Interpretation—visual field change should correspond to the optic disc appearance

1. Generalized peripheral constrictions—This is a fairly late change in the glaucoma field and other factors such as aging, miosis and hazy media cause the same contraction; therefore, it is of little diagnostic value.

2. Isolated paracentral scotomas—Small islands of relative or absolute scotomas may be demonstrated within the Bjerrum area. These may be isolated in the paracentral region only a few degrees from fixation, especially on the nasal side. They are a characteristic change of glaucoma and are separate from and do not connect with the blind spot. Later these defects enlarge and connect with the blind spot to form the classical arcuate scotoma. This is an early visual field change.

3. Nasal depression and nasal step—This is an early glaucoma defect. The depression extends in the horizontal raphe and forms a step on the superior portion.

4. Enlargement of the blind spot—This is a nonspecific change and is an uncommon early finding in glaucoma.

5. Nerve fiber bundle defect—This is a defect coming from the blind spot in an arcuate region extending to the horizontal raphe on the nasal side of the visual field.
6. Baring of the blind spot—This may be present in glaucoma but is not characteristic unless it is associated with the nasal step. It is of little diagnostic value.
7. Terminal temporal field—Visual acuity of 20/20 may be retained until very close to the terminal vision of glaucoma. Thus visual acuity is not an indicator of glaucoma control. An end-result is often a small crescent of temporal peripheral vision which remains after all other areas are gone.

Armaly, M. F.: Ocular Pressure and Visual Fields. Arch. Ophthal. 81: 25, 1969.

Drance, S. M.: The Visual Field in Glaucoma: Current Status. Trans. Amer. Acad. Ophthal. Otolaryng. 78:301-303, 1974.

Harrington, D. O.: The Bjerrum Scotoma. Amer. J. Ophthal. 59:646, 1965.

Heilmann, K.: On the Reversibility of Visual Field Defects in Glaucomas. Trans. Amer. Acad. Ophthal. Otolaryng. 78:304-308, 1974.

LeBlanc, R. P. and Beckers, B.: Peripheral Nasal Field Defects. Amer. J. Ophthal. 72:415, 1971.

Gonioscopy

1. Technique
   A. Indirect lens—A mirror arrangement permits exploration of the anterior chamber angle (Goldmann, Allen-Thorpe and Zeiss lenses). The patient sits upright at the slit lamp. A topical anesthetic is applied and either methyl cellulose or tears are used to place the contact lens on the cornea. Slit lamp is focused on the mirror arrangement and the anterior chamber angle is examined. Increased pressure on the lens indents the central cornea and tends to open the angle more widely. The Goldmann lens gives an excellent view of a narrow angle, is easy to place in narrow palpebral apertures, but presses on the cornea and, since it is hand held, may be wearing on the examiner. With the Allen-Thorpe lens, all four angles may be viewed without turning the prism; it is held

in position by the lids, and little or no pressure is placed on the cornea. However, it is relatively fragile, presents a limited view in narrow angles, and is difficult to place in a narrow palpebral fissure.

B. Direct gonioscopy lens—The observer looks directly into the anterior chamber angle through a Koeppe type of contact lens. The patient is supine. A topical anesthetic is given and the Koeppe lens is placed on the front portion of the eye and filled with fluid. A Barkan gonioscopy light and gonioscopy microscope are used to examine the anterior chamber structures. The Koeppe type of lens has several advantages: By inserting two lenses simultaneously, a rapid comparison of each eye can be made; little cooperation is required from patient; if an operative procedure is anticipated, it gives the same view as needed at surgery; the position is comfortable for examiner and patient; the supine position widens the angle.

2. Interpretation
   A. Angle width
      (1) Grade 0—No angle structures visible, narrow angle, complete or partial closure (angle closure)
      (2) Grade 1—Unable to see posterior 1/2 trabecular meshwork, extremely narrow angle (probably capable of angle closure)
      (3) Grade 2—Part of Schlemm's canal is visible, moderate narrow angle (may be capable of angle closure)
      (4) Grade 3—Posterior portion of Schlemm's canal is visible, moderate open angle (incapable of angle closure)
      (5) Grade 4—Ciliary body is visible, open angle (incapable of angle closure)

Forbes, M.: Gonioscopy with Corneal Indentation. A Method for Distinguishing between Appositional Closure and Synechial Closure. Arch. Ophthal. 76:488, 1966.

Hoskins, H. D.: Interpretive Gonioscopy in Glaucoma. Invest. Ophthal. 11:97-102, 1972.

Shaffer, R. N.: Stereoscopic Manual of Gonioscopy. St. Louis, C. V. Mosby, 1970.

B. Deep anterior chamber angle—differential diagnosis
   (1) Due to changes of the lens
      a. Dislocation (see p. 92)
      b. Glaucoma capsulare
   (2) Due to changes in the uveal tract
      a. Iritis and iridocyclitis (see p. 88)
      b. Tumor (see p. 79)
      c. Essential iris atrophy (see p. 83)
      d. Congenital anomalies such as posterior embryotoxon or aniridia
      e. Degenerative conditions such as pigmentary glaucoma (see p. 69)
      f. Rubeosis iridis (see rubeosis iridis, p. 85)
      g. Leukemic infiltrates of iris
   (3) Due to trauma
      a. Massive hemorrhage into the anterior or posterior chamber (see p. 73)
      b. Iridodialysis or recessed chamber angle (see p. 71)
      c. Intraocular foreign body, such as iron, especially in iris
      d. Lens dislocation (see p. 92)
      e. Epithelial downgrowth
   (4) Following surgical procedures
      a. Alpha-chymotrypsin induced
      b. Postoperative narrow-angle glaucoma with trabecular damage
      c. Hyphema (see p. 73)
      d. Epithelial downgrowth
      e. Following surgery for retinal detachment
   (5) Sturge-Weber syndrome (see p. 52)
   (6) Thyrotropic exophthalmos
   (7) Retrobulbar pressure—infection, tumor, or hemorrhage
   (8) Steroid-induced glaucoma (see p. 70)
   (9) Elevated episcleral venous pressure—dilated episcleral vessels (see p. 72)
   (10) Keratitis as metaherpetic (see p. 88)
   (11) Congenital glaucoma (see p. 47)
   (12) Aphakia (see p. 16)
   (13) Normal variation

(14) Open-angle glaucoma
(15) Myopia
(16) Megalocornea or conical cornea including keratoconus

Becker, B., and Shaffer, R. N.: Diagnosis and Therapy of Glaucoma, 3rd ed. St. Louis, C. V. Mosby, 1970, pp. 225-249.

Fonken, H. A. and Ellis, P. P.: Leukemic Infiltrates of the Iris. Arch. Ophthal. 76:32, 1966.

Newell, F. W.: Ophthalmology, Principles and Concepts. St. Louis, C. V. Mosby, 1969.

Roy, F. H.: Ocular Differential Diagnosis, 2nd ed. Philadelphia, Lea & Febiger, 1975, pp. 271-272.

Weekers, R. and Delmarcelle, Y.: Pathogenesis of Intraocular Hypertension in Cases of Arteriovenous Aneurysm. Arch. Ophthal. 48: 338-343, 1952.

C. Narrow anterior chamber angle—differential diagnosis
(1) Normal variation
(2) Predisposition to angle closure (see p. 75)
(3) Anterior dislocation of the lens (see p. 92)
(4) Hypermetropia
(5) Spherophakia and microcornea (see p. 75)
(6) Postoperative intraocular surgery with leaking wound
(7) Choroidal detachment
(8) Pupillary block
(9) Loss of aqueous from ocular perforation or staphyloma
(10) Intumescent senile cataract
(11) Traumatic cataract with secondary lenticular swelling (see p. 90)
(12) Primary hyperplastic primary vitreous
(13) Peripheral anterior synechiae (see p. 33)

Newell, F. W.: Ophthalmology, Principles and Concepts. St. Louis, C. V. Mosby, 1969.

D. Irregular depth of the anterior chamber—differential diagnosis
(1) Partial dislocation of the lens (see p. 92)
(2) Tumor or cyst on iris or ciliary body (see p. 79)

(3) Peripheral anterior synechiae on one side of the chamber (see p. 33)
(4) Iris bombé or pupillary block (see p. 91)
(5) Ruptured lens capsule with swelling on one side (see p. 90)
(6) Anatomical narrowing superiorly
(7) Subacute angle-closure glaucoma
(8) Cyclodialysis or traumatic recession of chamber angle (see p. 71)

Newell, F. W.: Ophthalmology, Principles and Concepts. St. Louis, C. V. Mosby, 1969.

E. Peripheral anterior synechiae—adhesion of iris tissue across the anterior chamber structures in variable amounts; noted with gonioscopy
(1) Bridge corneoscleral trabecular meshwork to Schwalbe's line or anterior to Schwalbe's line (uncommon)
a. Essential atrophy of iris (see p. 83)
b. Iris bombé from occlusion of pupil (see p. 91)
c. Postoperative flat anterior chamber
d. Penetrating injury of the cornea
e. Local adhesion with ingrowth of epithelium into aphakic eye
f. Anterior chamber cleavage syndrome
1) Congenital central anterior synechiae (Peter's anomaly)
2) Rieger's syndrome—hypoplasia of anterior iris and posterior embryotoxon
3) Axenfeld's syndrome—prominent anterior displacement Schwalbe's line (posterior embryotoxon) and iridocorneal angle adhesions
g. Tumor of iris or ciliary body pushing iris into contact with cornea (see p. 79)
(2) Synechiae of iris limited to ciliary band, scleral spur, and trabecular meshwork (common)
a. Sequelae from angle-closure glaucoma (see p. 75)
b. Intraocular inflammation (see p. 88)

c. Neovascular glaucoma—rubeosis iridis with shrinkage of fibrovascular membrane (see p. 85)

Chandler, P. A. and Grant, W. M.: Lectures on Glaucoma. Philadelphia, Lea & Febiger, 1965, pp. 276-279.

Kolker, A. E. and Hetherington, J.: Becker-Shaffer's Diagnosis and Therapy of the Glaucomas, 3rd ed. St. Louis, C. V. Mosby, 1970, pp. 197-206.

Newell, F. W.: Ophthalmology, Principles and Concepts. St. Louis, C. V. Mosby, 1969.

Reese, A. B. and Ellsworth, R.: The Anterior Chamber Cleavage Syndrome. Arch. Ophthal. 75:307, 1966.

F. Neovascularization of anterior chamber angle—differential diagnosis (see p. 85 for treatment of neovascular glaucoma). New-formed vessels extending onto the trabecular meshwork

(1) Proximal vascular disease
- a. Aortic arch syndrome
- b. Carotid occlusive disease
- c. Carotid ligation
- d. Carotid cavernous fistula
- e. Cranial arteritis

(2) Ocular vascular disease
- a. Central retinal vein thrombosis
- b. Central retinal artery thrombosis

(3) Retinal diseases
- a. Diabetes mellitus
- b. Leber's miliary aneurysms
- c. Coats' disease
- d. Eales' disease
- e. Sickle-cell retinopathy
- f. Retinal hemangioma
- g. Persistent hyperplastic primary vitreous
- h. Retrolental fibroplasia
- i. Retinoblastoma
- j. Norrie's disease
- k. Retinal detachment
- l. Melanoma of choroid
- m. Glaucoma, chronic

(4) Iris tumors
  a. Melanoma
  b. Metastatic carcinoma
  c. Hemangioma
(5) Postinflammatory conditions
  a. Uveitis, chronic, especially with heterochromic iridocyclitis (see p. 89)
  b. Surgery for retinal detachment
  c. Fungus endophthalmitis
  d. Radiation

Roy, F. H.: Ocular Differential Diagnosis, 2nd ed. Philadelphia, Lea & Febiger, 1975, pp. 318-319.

Schulze, R. R.: Rubeosis Iridis. Amer. J. Ophthal. 63:487, 1967.

G. Blood in Schlemm's canal—differential diagnosis
  (1) Normal eye
  (2) Tetralogy of Fallot—increased venous pressure (see p. 72)
  (3) Carotid-cavernous sinus fistula (see p. 72)
  (4) Intraocular inflammation
  (5) Hypotony
  (6) Mediastinal tumors—increased venous pressure
  (7) Any other process which increases venous pressure

Newell, F. W.: Ophthalmology, Principles and Concepts. St. Louis, C. V. Mosby, 1969, p. 34.

Phelps, C. D., et al.: Blood Reflux into Schlemm's Canal. Arch. Ophthal. 88:625-631, 1972.

Roy, F. H.: Ocular Differential Diagnosis, 2nd ed. Philadelphia, Lea & Febiger, 1975, p. 288.

Suson, E. B. and Schultz, R. W.: Blood in Schlemm's Canal in Glaucoma Suspects. Arch. Ophthal. 81:808, 1969.

H. Pigmentation of trabecular meshwork
  (1) Grade 0—no pigment
  (2) Grade 1—minimum pigment
  (3) Grade 2—moderate pigment
  (4) Grade 3—heavy pigment
  (5) Grade 4—dark pigment band

I. Pigmentation of trabecular meshwork—differential diagnosis
   (1) In elderly individuals—inferior nasal or faint circumferential band
   (2) Pseudoexfoliation of lens with glaucoma—unilateral or bilateral (see p. 68), wavy undulation of pigment
   (3) Pigmentary glaucoma (see p. 69)—wavy undulation of pigment
   (4) Krukenberg's spindle without glaucoma
   (5) Malignant melanoma—one eye
   (6) Cyst of pigment layer of iris—unilateral, irregular depth of anterior chamber (see p. 79)
   (7) Previous intraocular operation—inflammation, or scattered hyphema, mostly in lower angle (see p. 73)
   (8) Nevus—dense, isolated patch
   (9) Open-angle glaucoma—patchy band, whole circumference (see p. 60)
   (10) Previous unilateral gamma irradiation for malignancy of nasal sinus
   (11) Diabetes mellitus
   (12) Ocular trauma

Bothman, L.: Glaucoma Following Irradiation. Arch. Ophthal. 23:1198, 1940.

Chandler, P. A. and Grant, W. M.: Lectures on Glaucoma. Philadelphia, Lea & Febiger, 1965, p. 90.

Duncan, T. E.: Krukenberg Spindles in Pregnancy. Arch. Ophthal. 91:355-358, 1974.

Roy, F. H.: Ocular Differential Diagnosis, 2nd ed. Philadelphia, Lea & Febiger, 1975, p. 286.

J. Secondary open-angle glaucoma
   (1) Due to changes of the lens
      a. Dislocation
      b. Intumescence
      c. Phacolytic or phaco-anaphylactic
      d. Glaucoma capsulare
   (2) Due to changes in the uveal tract
      a. Iritis and iridocyclitis (see anterior uveitis, p. 88)

b. Tumor (see p. 79)
c. Essential iris atrophy
d. Congenital anomalies such as posterior embryotoxon or aniridia
e. Degenerative conditions such as pigmentary glaucoma
f. Rubeosis iridis (see rubeosis iridis, p. 34)
g. Leukemic infiltrates of iris

(3) Due to trauma
a. Massive hemorrhage into the anterior or posterior chamber
b. Corneal or limbal laceration with iris prolapse into the wound
c. Iridodialysis or recessed chamber angle
d. Intraocular foreign body, such as iron, especially in iris
e. Rupture of lens capsule with lens swelling
f. Lens dislocation (see p. 92)
g. Epithelial downgrowth

(4) Following surgical procedures
a. Alpha-chymotrypsin induced
b. Postoperative narrow-angle glaucoma with trabecular damage
c. Hyphema
d. Epithelial downgrowth
e. Following retinal detachment surgery

(5) Sturge-Weber syndrome
(6) Thyrotropic exophthalmos
(7) Retrobulbar pressure—infection, tumor, or hemorrhage
(8) Steroid-induced glaucoma
(9) Elevated episcleral venous pressure—dilated episcleral vessels (see p. 72)
(10) Keratitis as metaherpetic
(11) Retinitis pigmentosa
(12) Epidemic dropsy—consumption of argemone oil
(13) Congenital glaucoma (see p. 47)

Kolker, A. E. and Hetherington, J.: Becker-Shaffer's Diagnosis and Therapy of Glaucoma, 3rd ed. St. Louis, C. V. Mosby, 1970, pp. 225-249.

Fonken, H. A. and Ellis, P. P.: Leukemic Infiltrates of the Iris. Arch. Ophthal. 76:32, 1966.

Weekers, R. and Delmarcelle, Y.: Pathogenesis of Intraocular Hypertension in Cases of Arteriovenous Aneurysm. Arch. Ophthal. 48: 338-343, 1952.

Tonography

1. Technique–An electronic Schiotz (indention) tonometer is connected to a continuous reading and recording graph. This instrument is placed on the anesthesized eye of the patient lying on his back and left in place for four minutes. From the softening of the eye, the outflow facility coefficient (C) may be calculated: $C = F/P_0 - P_V$. Outflow facility equals outflow per minute/pressure gradient.
2. Interpretation–C values with open-angle glaucoma are likely to be low. Those eyes with severe glaucoma have C values averaging 0.05, those with moderate glaucoma 0.11, and those with early glaucoma 0.18. Normal C value is greater than 0.20.

Wilensky, J. T., Podas, S. M. and Becker, B.: Prognostic Indicators in Ocular Hypertension. Arch. Ophthal. 91:200-202, 1974.

GLAUCOMA MEDICAL THERAPEUTIC MODALITIES

1. Miotics
   A. Cholinergic drugs–simulate the effect of acetylcholine at autonomic synapses or the neuroeffector junctions of the parasympathetic system

U.S.P. or N.F. Name	*Concentration*	*Duration of Miotic Action*	*Representative Drug*
Pilocarpine	0.5–10%	4–6 hr.	Almocarpine Cellucarpine Isopto Carpine Mi-Pilo P.V. Carpine Pilo B Pilocar Pilocel Pilofrin Pilomiotin Pilovisc
Carbachol	0.25–3.0%	4–6 hr.	Carbacel Carbamiotin Isopto Carbachol

B. Anticholinesterases–inhibit the hydrolysis of acetylcholine by the enzyme cholinesterase

U.S.P. or N.F. Name	*Concentration*	*Duration of Miotic Action*
Physostigmine (Eserine)[a] (Isopto Eserine)	0.25 –1.0 %	≅ 4 hours–days
Neostigmine[a]	3.0 –5.0 %	
Diisopropyl fluorophosphate[b] (DFP, Floropryl)	0.035–0.1 %	days to weeks
Echothiophate iodide[b] (Phospholine iodide)	0.06 –0.25%	
Demecarium bromide[b] (Humorsol)	0.125–0.25%	

[a] Reversible anticholinesterases

[b] Irreversible anticholinesterases (Pralidoxime chloride and atropine may counteract the effects of these agents)

C. Complications and side effects of strong miotics

(1) Systemic toxicity—nausea, abdominal cramps, diarrhea, generalized weakness, inhibition of hydrolysis of succinylcholine so that respiratory paralysis may occur if the two drugs are given together

(2) Local effects—plastic iritis with secondary posterior synechiae, iris cysts, surgical hyphema, possible anterior subcapsular cataract, pupillary block and angle-closure glaucoma secondary to intense miosis and ciliary congestion, retinal detachment, pain around the eyes due to orbicularis spasm, irreversible miosis

D. To counteract accommodative spasm

(1) Weaken the miotic to help decrease accommodative spasm.

(2) Change to an epinephrine product to decrease the miotic effect. Great caution must be taken so that epinephrine given to a patient with narrow-angle glaucoma does not precipitate angle-closure glaucoma.

(3) Add Neo-Synephrine 10% up to three times a day to give some pupillary dilatation and decrease the miosis.

(4) Fit the individual with two pairs of glasses: one pair for average refraction and the second for the peak of accommodative spasm when vision is very blurred.

(5) Change the miotics to Diamox for ocular control. There are some disadvantages to systemic medication for this primary ocular disease.

(6) Reassure the patient that he needs to continue the medication for this sight-threatening disease.

2. Epinephrine

A. Types

Epinephrine Complex	*Percent Solution*	*Percent Base*
Bitartrate	2.0	1.1
Borate	1.0	1.0
Hydrochloride	2.0	2.0

B. Action—Epinephrine lowers intraocular pressure approximately 30% and, combined with a carbonic anhydrase inhibitor, a 65% reduction in aqueous flow may be achieved. Full effect may take as long as 2 to 3 months. Epinephrine probably acts in two ways: (1) decreased aqueous production, (2) increased facility of outflow.

C. Representative drugs
   (1) Adrenatrate—epinephrine bitartrate
   (2) Epifrin—L-epinephrine HCl
   (3) Epitrate—epinephrine bitartrate
   (4) Eppy—epinephryl borate
   (5) Glaucon—levo-epinephrine
   (6) Lyophrin—epinephrine bitartrate
   (7) Mytrate—epinephrine bitartrate

D. Indications
   (1) Lensopathy—Miotics will decrease visual acuity, especially with posterior subcapsular cataract.
   (2) Accommodative factor—Miotics will cause accommodative spasm, with pain and discomfort around eyes, and myopia, especially in people younger than 50 years.
   (3) Open angle—Narrow angle may congest and cause angle-closure glaucoma.

E. Disadvantages—Occasional allergy and prolonged use may leave conjunctival and corneal deposits or madarosis. Drugs are contraindicated in narrow-angle glaucoma.

F. Warnings—Use cautiously in hypertensive, diabetic, hyperthyroid or cardiovascular patients.

3. Topical drug combinations for glaucoma
   A. Bonmiotin—pilocarpine and eserine
   B. E-Pilo—epinephrine bitartrate and pilocarpine
   C. Isopto P-E-S—pilocarpine and physostigmine
   D. Miocel—eserine and pilocarpine
   E. P-E—pilocarpine and epinephrine bitartrate

4. Hyperosmotic agents—By virtue of their ability to create an osmolar gradient between blood and aqueous, they produce a fall in intraocular pressure.

A. Types

U.S.P. or N.F. Name	*Dosage*	*Route*	*Onset/ duration of Action*	*Complications and Side Effects*
Glycerol (50%)	1-1.5 gm/ kg body wgt	Oral	10-30 min. 4-5 hr.	Nausea and vomiting; may produce hyperglycemia and glycosuria
Mannitol (20%)	1-2 gm/kg body weight 2.5-10 ml/ kg	Intravenous	30-60 min. 6 hr.	Warm solution if crystals present
Urea (30%)	1-2 gm/kg body wgt 2-7 ml/kg	Intravenous	30-45 min. 5-6 hr.	Headache Sloughing of underlying tissue after extravasation
Isosorbide (50%)	1-2 gm/kg 2-4 ml/kg	Intravenous	30-45 min. 5-6 hr.	Penetrates eye slowly
Alcohol (40-50%)	0.8-1.5 gm/ kg 2-3 ml/kg	Oral	10-30 min. 4-5 hr.	CNS effects

B. Side effects—headache, back pain, dehydration, nausea and vomiting, agitation, chest pain, pulmonary edema, diuresis, subdural hematoma, K deficiency

5. Carbonic anhydrase inhibitors—produce a 30% to 60% reduction in the formation of aqueous humor in man without evidence of an alteration in the facility of its outflow

A. Types

U.S.P. or N.F. Name	*Dosage*	*Onset/ duration of Action*	*Complications or Side Effects in Long-term Therapy*
Acetazolamide oral (Diamox)	125-250 mg one to four times daily	2 hr. 4-6 hr.	Paresthesias, GI discomfort, anorexia, ureteral colic and calculi, potassium depletion, metabolic acidosis (acetazolamide is a sulfon-
Acetazolamide intravenous (Diamox)	250-500 mg in 5-10 ml distilled water	5-10 min. 2 hr.	

			amide derivative and similarly may cause skin reactions and bone marrow suppression)
Dichlorphenamide oral (Daranide, Oratrol)	50 mg one to four times daily	30 min. 6 hr.	Similar, but potassium depletion a more serious problem.
Ethoxzolamide oral (Cardrase, Ethamide)	125 mg one to four times daily	2 hr. 5 hr.	Similar to acetazolamide
Methazolamide oral (Neptazane)	50 - 100 mg three times a day	2 hr. 4-6 hr.	Similar, but generalized malaise, fatigue and drowsiness may develop

B. Side effects—K deficiency, rash, fever, drowsiness, paresthesias, crystalluria, renal calculus, bone marrow depression, and anorexia

6. Failure of medical therapy which might lead to surgical therapy
   A. Progression of visual field defect
   B. Changes in optic nerve appearance
   C. Inability to maintain adequate intraocular pressure
   D. Development of drug resistance
   E. Drug toxicity—drug intolerance
   F. Patient's temperament, understanding, cooperation, economy

Ophthalmic Prescription Handbook, 2nd ed. California, E. J. Browning Medical Publisher, 1968.

Physicians' Desk Reference for Ophthalmology. Oradell, Medical Economics, 1973.

Drance, S. M., Bensted, M. and Schulzer, M.: Pilocarpine and Intraocular Pressure. Arch. Ophthal. 91:104-106, 1974.

Humphreys, J. A. and Holmes, J. H.: Systemic Effects Produced by Echothiophate Iodide in Treatment of Glaucoma. Arch. Ophthal. 69:737, 1963.

Roy, F. H., et al.: Irreversible Miosis Following Long-Term Echothiophate (Phospholine) Iodide Use. J. Pediat. Ophthal. 7:46-49, 1970.

GLAUCOMA SURGICAL THERAPEUTIC MODALITIES

1. Iridectomy
   A. Indications for peripheral iridectomy
      (1) Anatomical closure of the angle (angle closure)
      (2) Mixed glaucoma, i.e., narrow and open-angle glaucoma combined
      (3) Progressive narrowing of the anterior chamber angle, as with peripheral anterior synechiae or increase in size of lens
      (4) Inability to use miotics because of angle narrowness—poor control without these medications
   B. Indications for sector iridectomy
      (1) Inflammation of the eye, to hold the pupil open
      (2) Corneal scarring, for optical reasons
      (3) Beginning cataract
      (4) Possibility of postoperative miotics, so that the patient can see better through a large pupillary opening
      (5) Retinal disease
2. Filter procedure
   A. Types
      (1) External, as punch, trephine, or Scheie procedure
      (2) Internal, as cyclodialysis
   B. Indications
      (1) Maximum medical therapy with progressive disc and visual field changes, especially for open-angle glaucoma
      (2) Refusal of medication
      (3) Aphakia
   C. Possible complications
      (1) Flat anterior chamber with PAS, corneal damage, cataract and/or closure of filter
      (2) Hypotonia with cataract formation
      (3) Loss of vision with thin-walled bleb and endophthalmitis
3. Destructive procedures
   A. Types—cyclocryotherapy or cyclodiathermy. Freezing is currently thought to be more effective than diathermy

B. Indications
   (1) Uncontrolled after filter and maximum medical therapy
   (2) Blind painful eye with increased pressure (absolute glaucoma)
   (3) Neovascular glaucoma
   (4) Infantile glaucoma—postgoniotomy
   (5) Patient who refuses other forms of glaucoma surgery

C. Possible complications
   (1) Pain from procedure
   (2) Iridocyclitis
   (3) Hyphema
   (4) Phthisis bulbi
   (5) Conjunctival scarring

4. Goniotomy—needle knife used to sweep embryonic tissue from chamber angle
   A. Indications—congenital or juvenile glaucoma with incomplete control
   B. Possible surgical complications
      (1) Hyphema
      (2) Flat anterior chamber
      (3) Cataract and/or iridodialysis

5. Alcohol injection
   A. Indications—blind painful eye without tumor with a relative contraindication to enucleation
   B. Procedure
      (1) Topical anesthesia
      (2) 1 cc 2% Xylocaine retrobulbar—needle in place if good anesthetic in 5 min.—injection of absolute alcohol
      (3) Ptosis with anesthetic or major paralysis of extraocular muscles should delay procedure

INSTRUCTIONS FOR GLAUCOMA PATIENT

1. Emotions—nervousness and anxiety
   A. Chronic glaucoma—no proven effect

B. Acute angle-closure glaucoma—some cases precipitated by marital problems, death in family, business problems, or severe physical illness or injury

2. Activities
   A. Physical activity—vigorous activity slightly lowers the intraocular pressure
   B. Reading or close work—no effect except with pathological narrowing of chamber angle from miosis and accommodation to precipitate attack of narrow-angle glaucoma from relative pupillary block
   C. Work and everyday activities—no alteration except if visual handicap makes it necessary to alter activities for patient's safety

3. Food and drink
   A. Food—transient osmotic effect
   B. Drink
      (1) Large volumes of fluid—transient rise in pressure
      (2) Tea and coffee—no appreciable effect
      (3) Alcoholic beverages—transient lowering of intraocular pressure

4. Systemic blood pressure
   A. Rapid increase in blood pressure may cause transient increase in intraocular pressure
   B. Chronic elevated blood pressure—With a prompt lowering of blood pressure or a low blood pressure, the circulation to the optic nerve suffers and the nerve fibers become more susceptible to damage by the intraocular pressure

5. Medicine
   A. Topical medication
      (1) Angle-closure glaucoma may be induced by use of sympathomimetic or parasympatholytic agents in the predisposed eye
      (2) No effect on chronic open-angle glaucoma
   B. Systemic medications
      (1) No effect on chronic open-angle glaucoma
      (2) Patients with narrow-angle glaucoma, as farsighted persons who have abnormally shallow chambers, in-

cluding older people, have a greater chance of angle-closure glaucoma from the use of psychopharmacological agents, antihistamines, antispasmodics and medications for parkinsonism

Chandler, P. A. and Grant, W. M.: Lectures on Glaucoma. Philadelphia, Lea & Febiger, 1965, pp. 21-26.

Peczon, J. D. and Grant, W. M.: Sedatives, Stimulants, and Intraocular Pressure in Glaucoma. Arch. Ophthal. 72:178-188, 1964.

Peczon, J. D. and Grant, W. M.: Sedatives, Stimulants, and Intraocular Pressure. Arch. Ophthal. 73:495-501, 1965.

Whitworth, C. G. and Grant, W. M.: Use of Nitrate and Nitrite Vasodilators by Glaucomatous Patients. Arch. Ophthal. 71:492-496, 1964.

INFANTILE GLAUCOMA (primary congenital glaucoma) —increased intraocular pressure due to defective embryological development of the anterior segment of the eye

1. Prevalence and genetic pattern–60% diagnosed in the first six months and 80% before one year; 60% of all patients affected by this rare anomaly male and the disease bilateral in 75% of the cases
2. Signs–congenital glaucoma should be diagnosed as early as possible
   A. Early signs
      (1) Epiphora, photophobia and blepharospasm–These may be present several weeks before the corneal haziness or enlargement becomes obvious. Normalizing the tension will promptly decrease these signs.
      (2) Corneal edema (haziness)–This symptom brings congenital glaucomas to the physician's attention most often. The later the onset of corneal edema, the better the prognosis. Other causes of corneal haziness must be ruled out. See page 17 for differential diagnosis of corneal opacification in an infant.
      (3) Corneal enlargement–Most infant corneas measure under 10.5 mm horizontal corneal diameter. A mea-

surement over 12 mm coupled with tears in Descemet's membrane is diagnostic of congenital glaucoma. The myopia induced by the enlargement of the eye is partially neutralized by the flattening of the cornea.

(4) Tears in Descemet's membrane—These tears may be single or multiple, appearing as an elliptical glassy ridge on the posterior cornea. At first they may be seen in the peripheral cornea, running parallel to the limbus. Later, the horizontal meridian is involved above and below the visual axis. Frequently this will cause a sudden clouding of the cornea as fluid is driven into the cornea.

(5) Deep anterior chamber—The chamber is deep because of the stretching of the cornea and flattening of the iris.

(6) Cupping and atrophy of the optic disc—Glaucomatous cupping appears early and progresses rapidly with uncontrolled pressures. Asymmetry and cupping of the optic disc are important early signs of glaucoma.

B. Late signs—Late changes are due to progression of the early signs. The cornea enlarges and becomes hazier and more protuberant, with a deepening of the anterior chamber. The limbal enlargement may stretch the zonular fibers, resulting in iridodonesis and even subluxation of the lens. Because these eyes are easily traumatized, corneal ulcers, hyphemas and rupture of the globe are not uncommon. Phthisis bulbi may be the result of the long uncontrolled intraocular pressure of infantile glaucoma.

3. Examination under anesthesia

A. Intraocular pressure check—All general anesthetics have a tendency to lower the intraocular pressure up to 15 to 20 mm Hg. If the child's intraocular pressure is checked just as he loses the Bell's phenomenon, with the mask still in place, this will often be fairly accurate. Horizontal applanation tonometry is probably superior to Schiotz tonometry.

B. Horizontal corneal diameter—Normally an infant's cornea

measures about 10.5 mm. A measurement over 11.5 mm is suspect, and diameters over 12 mm with tears in Descemet's membrane are diagnostic of congenital glaucoma. Occasionally in advanced glaucoma, the horizontal diameter will be over 14 mm. Glaucoma in microphthalmic eyes gives a smaller corneal diameter.

C. Gonioscopy—A deep anterior chamber and a flat iris plane are fairly characteristic of congenital glaucoma. The angle is usually wider than 45 degrees. There is a flat insertion of the iris into the trabecular meshwork. The trabecular surface may glisten like cellophane.

D. Ophthalmoscopy—There is early pathological cupping. Corneal haze and the astigmatism make the fundus examination difficult. Sometimes, after removal of the corneal epithelium, the fundus can be seen with greater clarity with the diagnostic contact lens.

4. Treatment

A. Medical—Miotics are of little value in the treatment of infantile glaucoma. They are used preoperatively to keep the pupil small for goniotomy, as an interval medication between operations, and terminally to prolong vision in eyes on which surgery has failed. Epinephrine has been found to be of value in treatment of some patients. Carbonic anhydrase inhibitors are useful preoperatively; 5 to 10 mg/kg of Diamox every six hours is a safe dose for infants. Medical treatment has been successful with the transient elevation of pressure that accompanies congenital rubella.

B. Surgical—Infantile glaucoma is primarily a surgical problem. An elevated intraocular pressure should not be the only criterion for surgery; other things (corneal edema, corneal enlargement, tears in Descemet's membrane, and glaucomatous disc cupping) must be evaluated also. Goniotomy is the best procedure for infantile glaucoma. Goniopuncture is a technique for fistulization used primarily in eyes in which repeated goniotomies have failed to clear the cornea for definitive surgery by temporary reduction in pressure. Fistulization procedures are of little value in the treatment of infantile glaucoma. The incision should be kept small since ectatic areas (staphylomas) occur frequently. Trabeculectomy and trabeculotomy have been fairly effective but are still in the experimental stage in our hands. Cyclocryotherapy is somewhat effective in decreasing discomfort and reducing intraocular pressure for several weeks and months. The incidence of phthisis bulbi is extremely low with this type of therapy.

5. Prognosis—The earlier the diagnosis of glaucoma is made and pressure brought into control, the better the prognosis. Most infants go blind unless successful surgery is performed. With the use of goniotomy less than half of those with signs present at birth can be salvaged, whereas of those whose disease becomes manifest between 2 and 9 months over 80% can be arrested. Forty percent of patients have vision below 20/200.

Barkan, O.: Pathogenesis of Congenital Glaucoma. Amer. J. Ophthal. 40:1, 1955.

Hoskins, H. D. and Shaffer, R. N.: Evaluation Techniques for the Congenital Glaucomas, J. Pediat. Ophthal. 8:660, 1971.

Kolker, A. E. and Hetherington, J.: Becker-Shaffer's Diagnosis and Therapy of the Glaucomas, 3rd ed. St. Louis, C. V. Mosby, 1970.

Shaffer, R. N. and Weiss, D. I.: Congenital and Pediatric Glaucomas. St. Louis, C. V. Mosby, 1970.

Worst, J. G. F.: The Pathogenesis of Congenital Glaucoma. Springfield, Charles C Thomas, 1966.

ANIRIDIA WITH GLAUCOMA—congenital absence of all but the most peripheral parts of the iris with an elevated intraocular pressure

1. Characteristics
   A. Aniridia may or may not be associated with glaucoma.
   B. There is autosomal dominant inheritance with 50% occurrence.
   C. If aniridia occurs as a mutant, it is unlikely that siblings or descendants will carry this gene.
   D. Usually the defective iris is noted by the parents or

physician, not the signs and symptoms of an elevated intraocular pressure. Nystagmus occurs frequently regardless of the presence or absence of glaucoma.

E. Initially there are small axial lens opacities and later there may be considerable lens opacity.

F. On gonioscopy, the filtration area is covered by a stump of iris in proportion to the severity of the glaucoma.

(1) In aniridic eyes having slight or mild glaucoma, the angle may show the iris stroma covering or closely attached to the filtration portion of the trabecular meshwork for only 1/3 to 1/2 of the circumference of the angle. There may be gaps through which normal ciliary body, scleral spur and filtration angle are visible.

(2) In aniridic eyes having moderate to severe glaucoma, the filtration area is covered by a forward attachment of the iris stroma over most of angle.

(3) The ciliary processes are well exposed to view by gonioscopy. These usually appear normal in individuals who have not had eye operations.

G. The glaucoma may be progressive.

2. Treatment

A. The treatment of glaucoma associated with aniridia is primarily medical. The treatment of choice is a miotic drug such as pilocarpine. Epinephrine and Diamox or other carbonic anhydrase inhibitors may then be helpful. A treatment regimen similar to that for open-angle glaucoma may be used (see p. 60).

B. Surgical therapy is necessary if medical treatment has proven inadequate. This consists of a form of goniotomy in which the congenital anterior synechiae which cross the trabecular meshwork are sharply dissected away to clear the filtration portion of the trabecular meshwork. Hyphema following goniotomy may be greater than that after congenital glaucoma. Three or four goniotomies may be performed to control pressure.

C. Trephine, cyclodialysis, or cyclodiathermy may be used but rarely successfully. Filtration operation with scleral cautery may be complicated by vitreous loss. Cyclocryotherapy may be of value.

Barkan, O.: Goniotomy for Glaucoma Associated with Aniridia. Arch. Ophthal. 49:1-5, 1953.

Becker, S. C.: Clinical Gonioscopy: A Text and Stereoscopic Atlas. St. Louis, C. V. Mosby, 1972.

Chandler, P. A. and Grant, W. M.: Lectures on Glaucoma. Philadelphia, Lea & Febiger, 1965, pp. 345-353.

HEMANGIOMA OF THE LID WITH GLAUCOMA—increase in the intraocular pressure associated with hemangioma of the upper eyelid

1. Characteristics
   - A. Most frequently the hemangioma affects only one side of the head and the corresponding eye. It is usually with hemangioma of the upper lid that an open-angle type of glaucoma can occur.
   - B. Hemangiomas of the lid are frequently accompanied by hemangiomas in other parts of the body. If the brain is involved, the condition is known as Sturge-Weber syndrome. Convulsions and epilepsy are common with involvement of the occipital cortex. Homonymous hemianopia may occur. With hemangiomas in the brain and kidneys, life expectancy is decreased.
   - C. If onset occurs early in infancy, there may be increase in the horizontal corneal diameter, glaucomatous cupping of the optic disc, haziness of cornea, and breaks in Descemet's membrane of the cornea.
   - D. On gonioscopy there are no characteristic abnormalities. Hemangiomas of the choroid are best seen with indirect ophthalmoscopy; however, diagnosis is made by angiography. Compare involved with uninvolved fundus.
   - E. The stroma of the iris of the eye with glaucoma in association with hemangioma may be thinner and more homogeneous than the normal eye, giving the affected iris a dark appearance (hyperchromic heterochromia).

2. Treatment
   A. For cases appearing in late childhood or adulthood, the preferred treatment is usually topical pilocarpine and epinephrine.
   B. For patients with hemangioma and glaucoma at an early age, the aggressiveness of the therapy will depend in part on the life expectancy. If there is involvement of the brain and kidneys, the life expectancy is shorter and treatment might be more conservative. Medical therapy of miotics, epinephrine, and carbonic anhydrase inhibitors is usually tried initially. If medical control is inadequate, then goniotomy is the treatment of choice although it is not nearly so effective as with infantile glaucoma. Filtering operations occasionally have been successful, with peripheral iridectomy and cautery.

Barkan, O.: Goniotomy for Glaucoma Associated with Nevus Flammeus. Amer. J. Ophthal. 43:545-549, 1957.

Chandler, P. A. and Grant, W. M.: Lectures on Glaucoma. Philadelphia, Lea & Febiger, 1965, pp. 354-357.

Scheie, H. G.: Results of Peripheral Iridectomy with Scleral Cautery in Congenital and Juvenile Glaucoma. Arch. Ophthal. 69:13-33, 1963.

Shaffer, R. N. and Weiss, D. I.: Congenital and Pediatric Glaucoma. St. Louis, C. V. Mosby, 1970, pp. 60-67.

Susac, J. O., Smith, J. L. and Scelfo, R. J.: The "Tomato-Catsup" Fundus in Sturge-Weber Syndrome. Arch. Ophthal. 92:69-70, 1974.

CONGENITAL GLAUCOMA ASSOCIATED WITH CONGENITAL CATARACT

1. Characteristics
   A. There may be an increase in the horizontal corneal diameter, breaks in Descemet's membrane, and corneal edema. If the eye has been microphthalmic previously then it may progress to a normal horizontal corneal diameter. It is important to compare it to the size of the other eye.
   B. Cataracts may vary from an incomplete opacity to a total opacity.

2. Differential diagnosis
   A. Lowe's syndrome (oculocerebrorenal syndrome)—systemic acidosis, organic aciduria, decreased ability to produce ammonia in the kidneys, renal rickets, generalized hypotonicity, mental retardation, and congenital glaucoma
   B. Congenital rubella syndrome – deafness, retinopathy, thrombocytopenia, cardiac defects
   C. Hallerman-Streiff syndrome—dyscephaly, birdlike facies, proportionate nanism, localized hypotrichosis, localized atrophy of skin, bilateral microphthalmia, and congenital glaucoma
   D. Trisomy 16-18—failure to thrive, low-set ears, malformed pinnae, mental retardation, hypertonicity, small mouth and mandible, ventricular septal defects, optic atrophy, and congenital glaucoma
   E. Garlin-Goltz syndrome (multiple basal cell nevi syndrome)—glaucoma, strabismus, hypertelorism
   F. Turner syndrome (male)—myopia, retinal detachment and glaucoma
   G. Pierre Robin syndrome—hypoplasia of the mandible, glossoptosis, cleft palate, high myopia, retinal detachment, glaucoma, cataracts, and microphthalmia
   H. Idiopathic infantile hypoglycemia—neonatal hypoglycemia, nasolacrimal duct obstructions, congenital cataracts, squint, cortical blindness, atrophy of the optic disc, congenital glaucoma

3. Treatment
   A. Control of intraocular pressure, as with open-angle infantile glaucoma (see p. 47)
   B. Cataract surgery on the affected eye at a later date, if sufficient lens opacity

Chandler, P. A. and Grant, W. M.: Lectures on Glaucoma. Philadelphia, Lea & Febiger, 1965, pp. 358-363.

Roy, F. H.: Ocular Differential Diagnosis, 2nd ed. Philadelphia, Lea & Febiger, 1975, pp. 268-269, 343-346.

Wilson, W. A., Richards, W., and Donnell, G. N.: Oculo-cerebral-renal syndrome of Lowe. Arch. Ophthal. 70:5-11, 1963.

RETROLENTAL FIBROPLASIA WITH GLAUCOMA

1. Characteristics
   A. There is a retrolental membrane (see #2 below for differential diagnosis of leukokoria). This may be confused with retinoblastoma. A white membrane is posterior to or involving the posterior capsule of the lens.
   B. The anterior chamber characteristically is shallow.
   C. Age of onset may be from a few months of birth to early childhood. Onset is usually acute, with pain in the eye, nausea and vomiting. With gonioscopy, an angle-closure glaucoma is apparent.
   D. Segmental atrophy of the iris stroma may occur.
   E. History of low birth weight, respiratory distress and incubator oxygen is frequently given.

2. Differential diagnosis of leukokoria
   A. Retinoblastoma
   B. Cataract (congenital)
   C. Nematode endophthalmitis (*Toxocara canis*)
   D. Coats' disease
   E. Persistent hyperplastic primary vitreous
   F. Retrolental fibroplasia
   G. Retinal dysplasia (massive retinal fibrosis)
   H. Vitreous organization following unsuspected penetrating wounds
   I. Organized vitreous hemorrhage
   J. Falciform fold of retina
   K. Angiomatosis of retina
   L. Retrolental membrane associated with Bloch-Sulzberger syndrome (incontinentia pigmenti)
   M. Exudative retinitis or chorioretinitis or both
   N. Diktyoma
   O. Congenital retinal detachment
   P. Norrie's disease
   Q. Juvenile retinoschisis
   R. Metastatic endophthalmitis
   S. Tumors other than retinoblastoma

T. Coloboma of choroid and optic disc
U. Medullation of nerve fiber layer
V. Traumatic chorioretinitis
W. High myopia with advanced chorioretinal degeneration

3. Treatment
   A. The degree of impairment of vision from traction of the macula and disc to the retrolental membrane, cataract, and retinal separation must be taken into consideration in terms of treatment.
   B. The disease should be treated similarly to acute angle-closure glaucoma, by lowering the intraocular pressure and performing a peripheral iridectomy (see p. 75).
   C. In an eye that is essentially blind before onset of glaucoma, the pain sometimes can be controlled medically with aspirin, carbonic anhydrase inhibitors, etc. Cyclocryotherapy or alcohol injection may be considered. At a later time, the pressure may subside and the globe become atrophic and painless.
   D. Sometimes enucleation is necessary in a blind, painful eye.

Chandler, P. A. and Grant, W. M.: Lectures on Glaucoma. Philadelphia, Lea & Febiger, 1965, pp. 364-366.

Gitter, K. A., Meyer, D., White, R. H., Ortolon, G., and Sarin, L. K.: Ultrasonic Aid in the Evaluation of Leukokoria. Amer. J. Ophthal. 65:190, 1968.

Hansen, A. C.: Norrie's Disease. Amer. J. Ophthal. 66:328-332, 1968.

Hogan, M. F. and Zimmerman, L. E.: Ophthalmic Pathology, 2nd ed. Philadelphia, W. B. Saunders, 1962, p. 523.

Howard, G. M. and Ellsworth, R. M.: Differential Diagnosis of Retinoblastoma: A Statistical Survey of 500 Children. Amer. J. Ophthal. 60:610, 1965.

Jones, S. T.: Retrolental Membrane Associated with Bloch-Sulzberger Syndrome (Incontinentia Pigmenti). Amer. J. Ophthal. 62:330, 1966.

Roy, F. H.: Ocular Differential Diagnosis, 2nd ed. Philadelphia, Lea & Febiger, 1975, pp. 310-311.

GLAUCOMA SECONDARY TO OPERATION FOR CONGENITAL CATARACTS

1. Prevention—Many cases could be avoided. The formation of an inflammatory membrane, posterior synechiae, pupillary block, peripheral anterior synechiae, and glaucoma is the usual course following congenital cataract. Prevention, then, takes four different courses.
   A. The postoperative use of atropine for several months after surgery until there is a complete clearing of the anterior chamber inflammation
   B. Iris surgery to open the pupil as a sector iridectomy above with a sphincterotomy at 9, 6 and 3 o'clock
   C. Removal of as much of the anterior capsule and lens material as possible to cut down on inflammation following surgery
   D. Steroids to reduce inflammation in the anterior chamber. If the lenses are congenitally dislocated, see glaucoma associated with dislocation of the lens, page 92. If glaucoma results from inflammation following a perforating injury, see page 88.

2. Early signs of pupillary block and glaucoma
   A. Characteristics—Iris bombé, an overall shallowing of the anterior chamber, unevenness in depth of the anterior chamber or peripheral anterior synechiae extending onto clear cornea
   B. Treatment—Vigorous; if unsuccessful, however, an iridectomy may be necessary

3. Late signs of pupillary block and glaucoma
   A. Characteristics – Glaucoma sometimes is diagnosed promptly after pupillary block has developed, but many cases are diagnosed late. In an infant, the eye may become enlarged with an increased horizontal corneal diameter, corneal edema and photophobia. The intraocular pressure will be increased and there will be glaucomatous changes of the optic nerve heads. In many cases the glaucoma is discovered several years after operation on congenital cataract because of nystagmus and the poor

pupillary opening. The severity of the glaucoma is usually approximately equal to the amount of angle obstructed by peripheral anterior synechiae.

B. Treatment—The standard antiglaucoma medications are tried to see if the glaucoma can be controlled medically (see p. 60). If medical control fails, surgery is usually tried: a filtering operation initially, followed by cyclodialysis or cryotherapy. Control of this type of glaucoma in children is very difficult, and the eye may be lost.

Chandler, P. A. and Grant, W. M.: Lectures on Glaucoma. Philadelphia, Lea & Febiger, 1965, pp. 367-375.

Shaffer, R. N. and Weiss, D. I.: Congenital and Pediatric Glaucomas. St. Louis, C. V. Mosby, 1970, pp. 169-172.

XANTHOGRANULOMA WITH SECONDARY GLAUCOMA

1. Characteristics
   - A. Spontaneous hemorrhage in the anterior chamber may or may not be associated with a yellow mass or nodules of the iris. It is important to look at a differential diagnosis of spontaneous hyphema in an infant (see #2 below).
   - B. With glaucoma there may be pain in the eye, edema of the cornea, enlargement of the cornea with breaks in Descemet's membrane and blood staining of the cornea.
   - C. Skin lesions of a yellowish macular papular nature may be present on the skin.
   - D. If possible, clinical diagnosis is confirmed by biopsy of skin or epibulbar lesion. Biopsy of iris would infrequently be indicated. Anterior chamber paracentesis may be of value.
2. Differential diagnosis of spontaneous hyphema in infant
   - A. Juvenile xanthogranuloma
   - B. Retinoblastoma
   - C. Blood dyscrasias such as anemia and leukemia
   - D. Acute rheumatoid iridocyclitis
   - E. Trauma without history

F. Retrolental fibroplasia
G. Persistent hyperplastic vitreous
H. Retinoschisis
I. Iritis

3. Treatment
   A. Treatment with corticosteroids topically and systemically
   B. X-radiation (150 to 200 r, not exceeding a total dose of 450-500 r) to shrink the iris lesions
   C. Carbonic anhydrase inhibitors to lower the intraocular pressure

Duke-Elder, S. and Perkins, E. S.: Diseases of the Uveal Tract. System of Ophthalmology, Vol. IX. St. Louis, C. V. Mosby, 1966, pp. 19-20.

Gass, J. D.: Management of Juvenile Xanthogranuloma of the Iris. Arch. Ophthal. 71:344-347, 1964.

Guzak, S. V.: Lymphoma as a Cause of Hyphema. Arch. Ophthal. 84: 229-231, 1970.

Howard, G. M.: Spontaneous Hyphema in Infancy and Childhood. Arch. Ophthal. 68:615-620, 1962.

Roy, F. H.: Ocular Differential Diagnosis, 2nd ed. Philadelphia, Lea & Febiger, 1975, p. 285.

Shaffer, R. N. and Weiss, D. I.: Congenital and Pediatric Glaucomas. St. Louis, C. V. Mosby, 1970, pp. 144-149.

Schwartz, L. W., Rodrigues, M. M., and Hallett, J. W.: Juvenile Xanthogranuloma Diagnosed by Paracentesis. Amer. J. Ophthal. 77:243-247, 1974.

JUVENILE OPEN-ANGLE GLAUCOMA—This is the same as open-angle glaucoma in adults, except that it has an earlier onset, in childhood or adolescence. Intraocular pressure is elevated and an open-angle chamber angle is revealed by gonioscopy.

1. Characteristics
   A. Open-angle gonioscopy. The course of the disease can be divided into four different types, as open-angle glaucoma (see p. 60), in terms of ocular hypertension, early glaucoma, moderate glaucoma, or severe glaucoma. The treatment can be managed in the same way
   B. Many times asymptomatic, as open-angle glaucoma

C. Autosomal dominant trait

2. Treatment
   A. With a positive family history, early recognition is important. It is important that the individual be checked starting at an early age, with tonometry and examination of the optic nerve disc. Relatives and siblings should be examined.
   B. Treatment is the same as that for open-angle glaucoma (see p. 60). If miotics are necessary, the stronger, longer-acting miotics are usually preferable, in that the degree of induced myopia is more constant and therefore more satisfactorily corrected with glasses. However, these drugs may induce lens changes and should be used with caution.
   C. If the glaucoma is diagnosed early, epinephrine is preferable to miotics in controlling the pressure.
   D. Carbonic anhydrase inhibitor drugs are not usually used for long-term therapy because of the undesirable side effects.
   E. Filtering operation would be the procedure of choice if medical therapy does not control the condition.

Chandler, P. A. and Grant, W. M.: Lectures on Glaucoma. Philadelphia, Lea & Febiger, 1965, pp. 378-380.

Scheie, H. G.: Results of Peripheral Iridectomy with Scleral Cautery in Congenital and Juvenile Glaucoma. Arch. Ophthal. 69:13-33, 1963.

OPEN-ANGLE GLAUCOMA—an elevated intraocular pressure and an open anterior chamber angle by gonioscopy. Four clinical types are apparent in this continuous spectrum of abnormalities. Open-angle glaucoma is primarily a medical disease

1. Ocular hypertension
   A. Characteristics—The cup/disc ratio is 0.3 or lower with no asymmetry between each disc. The fields are within normal limits. The intraocular pressures are elevated, above 21 mm Hg applanation or 23 mm Hg Schiotz.

B. Management

(1) The individual is examined every 6 months for changes in the optic disc and visual fields.

(2) With a family history of glaucoma, blindness, high myopia, large or deep cups, anemia, hypotension, only eye, or a patient history of diabetes or vascular disease, the individual would be followed more frequently and might be classed as an early glaucoma and treated.

(3) If the pressure is over 30 mm Hg, pilocarpine 1% or epinephrine may be tried. If there is excellent reduction of pressure and minimum discomfort to the patient, the eye will probably be safer at 18 than 28 mm Hg. The patient then can be maintained on this medication. If, however, there is considerable discomfort from pilocarpine and there is no significant drop in pressure, then it might be feasible to permit that patient to remain at a pressure higher than the statistically normal, instead of prescribing stronger medication, until such time that there is a change in the optic cup or loss of visual field.

2. Early glaucoma

A. Characteristics—There is a cup/disc ratio of 0.4 to 0.5, a cup that is vertically oval, or a cup that extends upward or downward to touch the margin of the disc with the visual fields demonstrating isolated paracentral scotomas, nasal depression and nasal step, or nerve fiber bundle defect.

B. Management—The first 6 to 8 weeks of therapy should lower the intraocular pressure below 24 mm Hg, the maintenance level. The patient should be brought back every 1 to 2 weeks to determine if a satisfactory drop in intraocular pressure toward the maintenance level has occurred. If not, the following stepwise increase in therapy may be followed:

(1) If the patient is young and might have accommodative spasm, either pilocarpine 1/2 to 1% four times a day or epinephrine 1% twice a day would be started.

The intraocular pressure would be rechecked in 1 or 2 weeks to see if there had been a suitable drop. If not, the following stepwise increase in therapy is followed (NOTE: consider higher concentrations of drugs in dark iris):

a. Pilocarpine 1/2 to 1% q.i.d. or epinephrine 1% b.i.d.
b. Pilocarpine 2% q.i.d.
c. Pilocarpine 4% q.i.d.
d. Pilocarpine 4% q.i.d. and epinephrine 1% b.i.d.
e. Pilocarpine 4% q.i.d., epinephrine 1% b.i.d., and Diamox 250 mg up to four times a day
f. Phospholine iodide up to 0.25% b.i.d., epinephrine 1% b.i.d. and Diamox 250 mg up to four times a day. This is maximum medical therapy
g. Surgery for glaucoma
   1) Filtering procedure
   2) Cryocyclodiathermy or cyclodiathermy

(2) If the individual is older, 2% pilocarpine four times a day would be started and the individual asked to return in 1 to 2 weeks to see if there has been a suitable drop in intraocular pressure. If posterior subcapsular cataracts are present, epinephrine may be started instead. If not, the following stepwise increase in therapy is followed:

a. Pilocarpine 2% q.i.d.
b. Pilocarpine 4% q.i.d.
c. Pilocarpine 4% q.i.d. and epinephrine 1% b.i.d.
d. Pilocarpine 4% q.i.d., epinephrine 1% b.i.d. and Diamox 250 mg up to four times a day
e. Phospholine iodide up to 0.25% b.i.d., epinephrine 1% b.i.d. and Diamox 250 mg up to four times a day (maximum medical therapy)
f. Surgery for glaucoma
   1) Filtering procedure
   2) Cryocyclodiathermy or cyclodiathermy
   3) Cyclodialysis

Usually with an early glaucoma, the intraocular pressure should be held below 24 mm Hg for a maintenance level. If, however, there was a loss of the visual field, then an increase in therapy should be entertained even with no change in the cup/disc ratio. As a general rule, the smaller the cup, the better the eye withstands an increased intraocular pressure.

3. Moderate glaucoma
   A. Characteristics–The disc has a cup/disc ratio of 0.6 to 0.7 and visual field changes might consist of isolated paracentral scotomas, nasal depression and nasal step, enlargement of the blind spot, nerve fiber bundle defect, and baring of the blind spot. On tonogram the C value would be 0.15 or less.
   B. Management–The first 6 to 8 weeks of therapy should lower the intraocular pressure below 20 mm Hg, the maintenance level. The patient should be brought back every 1 to 2 weeks to determine if a satisfactory drop in intraocular pressure toward the maintenance level has occurred. If not, the following stepwise increase in therapy is followed:
      (1) Pilocarpine 2% q.i.d.
      (2) Pilocarpine 4% q.i.d.
      (3) Pilocarpine 4% q.i.d., and epinephrine 1% b.i.d.
      (4) Pilocarpine 4% q.i.d., epinephrine 1% b.i.d., and Diamox 250 mg up to four times a day
      (5) Phospholine iodide up to 0.25% b.i.d., epinephrine 1% b.i.d. and Diamox 250 mg up to four times a day. This is maximum medical therapy
      (6) Surgery for glaucoma
         a. Filtering procedure
         b. Cryocyclodiathermy or cyclodiathermy
         c. Cyclodialysis

4. Severe glaucoma
   A. Characteristics–Cup/disc ratio is 0.8 or larger and the visual field defects include a generalized peripheral constriction, nasal depression and nasal step, enlargement of

the blind spot and a terminal temporal visual field. The tonogram will demonstrate a C value of 0.15 or less. Poor discs do not tolerate much pressure elevation.

B. Management—The first 6 to 8 weeks of therapy should lower the intraocular pressure to an acceptable level. The goal is to maintain the intraocular pressure below 18 mm Hg. There are two ways in which this problem can be managed:

(1) Stepwise increase in medical therapy at 1- to 2-week intervals
   a. Pilocarpine 2% q.i.d.
   b. Pilocarpine 4% q.i.d.
   c. Pilocarpine 4% q.i.d. and epinephrine 1% b.i.d.
   d. Pilocarpine 4% q.i.d., epinephrine 1% b.i.d. and Diamox 250 mg up to four times a day
   e. Phospholine iodide up to 0.25% b.i.d., epinephrine 1% b.i.d. and Diamox 250 mg up to four times a day
   f. Glaucoma surgery, as filtering procedure or cryo-cyclodiathermy

(2) Start maximum medical therapy of Phospholine iodide, epinephrine 1% b.i.d. and Diamox 250 mg q.i.d., and have patient return in two weeks. If there has been a satisfactory decrease in intraocular pressure, the medication can be slowly withdrawn until a maintenance level below 18 mm Hg is obtained

5. Open-angle glaucoma and cataracts

A. Reassure patient and try to control pressure with epinephrine and carbonic anhydrase inhibitors rather than miotics.

B. Control the pressure preoperatively, perform cataract extraction, then continue medication postoperatively as needed.

C. Treat uncontrolled tension by:

(1) Filtering operation initially and cataract extraction at later date
(2) Cataract extraction and cyclodialysis
(3) Cataract extraction and filtering operation

Baloglon, P., Matta, C., and Asdourian, K.: Cataract Extraction After Filtering Operations. Arch. Ophthal. 88:12-15, 1972.

Bigger, J. F. and Becker, B.: Cataracts and Primary Open-Angle Glaucoma. Trans. Amer. Acad. Ophthal. Otolaryng. 75:260-272, 1971.

Chandler, P. A. and Grant, W. M.: Lectures on Glaucoma. Philadelphia, Lea & Febiger, 1965, pp. 109-142.

Johnson, S. B.: Combined Cataract Extraction and Scleral Cautery. Ann. Ophthal. 3:1163-1166, 1971.

Morgan, R. W.: Open-Angle Glaucoma: An Epidemiologist's View. Canad. J. Ophthal. 7:75-79, 1972.

Randolph, E., Maumenee, E., and Iliff, C.: Cataract Extraction in Glaucomatous Eyes. Amer. J. Ophthal. 71:328-330, 1971.

Regan, E. F. and Day, R. M.: Cataract Extraction After Filtering Procedures. Amer. J. Ophthal. 71:331-334, 1971.

Sugar, H. S.: Principles of Medical Management in Chronic Open Angle Glaucoma. Ann. Ophthal. 3:579, 1971.

Sugar, H. S.: The Surgical Treatment of Chronic Open-Angle Glaucoma. Amer. J. Ophthal. 59:656-668, 1965.

LOW-TENSION GLAUCOMA—intraocular pressure at all times below 22 mm Hg by Goldmann applanation tonometer but progressive cupping and atrophy of the optic nerve and loss of field as with open-angle glaucoma

1. Characteristics
   A. Condition occurs in older individuals.
   B. Both eyes are affected in a similar manner.
   C. Intraocular pressure is lower than 18 to 19 mm Hg and the facility is at lower end of normal (C 0.20).
   D. In some cases the above measurements become worse and the diagnosis changes from low-tension to open-angle glaucoma.
   E. Likely to have hemodynamic crisis, low systemic blood pressure or low ophthalmic blood pressure.
2. Differential diagnosis—With glaucomatous cupping and a normal intraocular pressure, other possibilities must be ruled out. Most cases are *not* low-tension glaucoma. Helpful information

may be obtained from applanation tonometry every 3 to 4 hours day and night, tonography, water-drinking by tonography, and neurologic examination.

A. Primary open-angle glaucoma with large diurnal variation and elevation of intraocular pressure above 22 mm Hg at some time of the day or night (see p. 60)
B. Decreased scleral rigidity with Schiotz intraocular pressure but elevated Goldmann applanation pressure as with myopia, thyroid exophthalmos, after ocular surgery, use of strong miotics as Phospholine iodide, and water drinking
C. Previously elevated intraocular pressures which are now normal, previous intraocular inflammation as anterior or posterior synechiae and pigmented old inflammatory deposits, previous use of corticosteroids causing transient elevation of intraocular pressure
D. Congenital anomalies of the optic disc
   (1) Oblique insertion of the optic nerve
   (2) Branching of vessels behind the lamina, so that individual branches appear at the disc margins
   (3) Congenital coloboma of the disc
   (4) Coloboma within the nerve sheath
   (5) Traction of the disc with bowing of the scleral crescent
E. Sclerosis or calcification of the internal carotid arteries with pressure on optic nerves or arteriosclerosis of the nutrient vessels of the optic nerve
F. Tumors arising near the chiasm (rare)
G. Syphilitic optic atrophy
H. Open-angle glaucoma with hyposecretion of aqueous and decreased facility of outflow—diagnosed by tonography (see p. 60)
I. "Weak" optic disc which atrophies at normal pressures or reduced blood pressure to optic nerve, as severe blood loss, gastrointestinal bleeding, acute hypotension, myocardial infarction, carotid insufficiency, or nutritional deficiencies
J. Schnabel's cavernous atrophy

K. Digitalis therapy

L. Cerebral atrophy and status lacunaris

3. Treatment—Without treatment, even with low intraocular pressure, defects in the visual field and cupping of the optic nerve may progress as those in primary open-angle glaucoma. Changes in the optic disc may be progressive because of defective circulation of the optic nerve heads, low systemic blood pressures, and/or pernicious anemia.
   A. Rule out other causes of cupping and atrophy of optic disc and field loss (see differential diagnosis above).
   B. Moderate to heavy antiglaucoma medications may reduce tension. Usually medical therapy has little effect on intraocular pressure.
   C. In very old individuals, if the progressive changes will not cause complete loss of vision during the probable lifetime, vigorous medical therapy may maintain sufficiently slow visual loss.
   D. In younger individuals where changes are progressive, filtering operation, especially trephine, may be necessary to get the pressure as low as possible.

Chandler, P. A.: Long-Term Results in Glaucoma Therapy. Amer. J. Ophthal. 49:221-246, 1960.

Chandler, P. A. and Grant, W. M.: Lectures on Glaucoma. Philadelphia, Lea & Febiger, 1965, pp. 143-146.

Deutsch, A. R.: Differential Characteristics of Low Tension Glaucoma. J. Tenn. Med. Assoc. 54:84-89, 1961.

Drance, S. M.: Some Factors in the Production of Low Tension Glaucoma. Brit. J. Ophthal. 56:229-242, 1972.

Drance, S. M., et al.: Studies of Factors Involved in the Production of Low Tension Glaucoma. Arch. Ophthal. 89:457-465, 1973.

Hiatt, R. L., Deutsch, A. R., and Ringer, C.: Low Tension Glaucoma. Ann. Ophthal. 3:85-92, 1971.

Leighton, D. A. and Phillips, C. I.: Systemic Blood Pressure in Open-Angle Glaucoma, Low Tension Glaucoma, and the Normal Eye. Brit. J. Ophthal. 56:447-453, 1972.

McDonald, T. J.: Problems of Low Tension Glaucoma. Trans. Ophthal. Soc. U. K. 87:873-892, 1967.

OPEN-ANGLE GLAUCOMA ASSOCIATED WITH LENS CAPSULE PSEUDOEXFOLIATION

1. Characteristics
   A. Open angle with elevated intraocular pressure—most frequent in older individuals with nuclear sclerosis; chamber may be narrowed
   B. Frequently excessive pigmentation of trabecular meshwork, back surface of the cornea and front surface of the iris
   C. Transillumination of the iris revealing patchy loss of pigment from the posterior pigment layer adjacent to the pupil
   D. Pseudoexfoliation material at the pupillary border and face of the lens. Fine light gray amorphous flakes which resemble dandruff may be present at the pupillary margin. A lusterless gray membrane covers the pupillary area of the anterior lens capsule which ends under the iris in a series of scallops peripherally and sometimes a curled edge on the anterior surface of the lens
   E. Gradual development into chronic and permanent state, increasing in severity with time
   F. Unilaterality in 65% of cases
   G. Geographic distribution—Scandinavia, Bantu and west coast of United States.

2. Treatment
   A. Medical therapy as for open-angle glaucoma (see p. 61)
   B. Control with miotics and epinephrine more difficult than in open-angle glaucoma
   C. Surgical therapy as for open-angle glaucoma (see p. 63)
   D. Cataract extraction useless to control intraocular pressure. When antiglaucoma surgery and cataract extraction are both needed, the same principles as in open-angle glaucoma and cataract are applied (see p. 64)

Becker, S. C.: Clinical Gonioscopy. St. Louis, C. V. Mosby, 1972, pp. 124-127.

Chandler, P. A. and Grant, W. M.: Lectures on Glaucoma. Philadelphia, Lea & Febiger, 1965, pp. 147-149.

Gillies, W. E.: Racial Incidence of Pseudo-Exfoliation of the Lens Capsule. Brit. J. Ophthal. 56:474-477, 1972.

Lantz, M. H.: Prevalence of Pseudo-Exfoliation Syndrome in an Urban South African Clinic Population. Amer. J. Ophthal. 74:581-587, 1972.

Layden, W. E. and Shaffer, R. N.: The Exfoliation Syndrome. Trans. Amer. Acad. Ophthal. Otolaryng. 78:326-327, 1974.

Pohjarpelta, P. and Hurskoiuen, L.: Studies on Relatives of Patients with Glaucoma Simplex and Patients with Pseudo-Exfoliation of the Lens Capsule. Acta Ophthal. 50:255-261, 1972.

PIGMENTARY GLAUCOMA—bilateral elevated intraocular pressure, open angle gonioscopically, and a heavy accumulation of dark brown pigment in the whole circumference (several observers question this entity)

1. Clinical characteristics
   - A. Moderate myopia with some astigmatism
   - B. Pigment dispersion
     - (1) Loss of pigment epithelium from the periphery and midperiphery of the iris by retroillumination
     - (2) Pigment deposition on posterior corneal surface (Krukenberg spindle)
     - (3) Pigment deposition on trabecular meshwork
     - (4) Pigment deposition on anterior iris and lens
   - C. Same course as open-angle glaucoma (see p. 60)—chronic and insidious
   - D. Intraocular pressure lowered with pilocarpine and elevated with mydriasis, without any narrowness of chamber angle
   - E. More frequent in males and middle-aged individuals (20 to 45 years)
   - F. Wide swings in intraocular pressure—decreased severity with time

2. Treatment
   - A. Medical treatment same as that for open-angle glaucoma (see p. 61)
   - B. Surgical treatment same as that for open-angle glaucoma (see p. 63)

Chandler, P. A. and Grant, W. M.: Lectures on Glaucoma. Philadelphia, Lea & Febiger, 1965, pp. 150-155.

Lichter, P. R.: Pigmentary Glaucoma—Current Concepts. Trans. Amer. Acad. Ophthal. Otolaryng. 78:309-313, 1974.

Lichter, P. R. and Shaffer, R. N.: Diagnostic and Prognostic Signs in Pigmentary Glaucoma. Trans. Amer. Acad. Ophthal. Otolaryng. 74: 984-999, 1970.

Perkins, E. S. and Joy, B. S.: Pigmentary Glaucoma. Trans. Ophthal. Soc. U. K. 80:153, 1960.

Sugar, H. S.: Pigmentary Glaucoma: A 25 Year Review. Amer. J. Ophthal. 62:499-507, 1966.

CORTICOSTEROID GLAUCOMA—increase in intraocular pressure in open-angle eye after topical administration of corticosteroids

1. Characteristics
   - A. Relatives of patients with open angle may have dramatic increase in tension with use of topical corticosteroids.
   - B. Administration of topical corticosteroids aggravates control of open-angle glaucoma.
   - C. Condition may lead to cupping and atrophy of optic nerve head with extensive loss of visual fields.
   - D. Patient may be using steroids for ocular disease as chronic uveitis, blepharitis or conjunctivitis.
2. Treatment
   - A. Discontinue corticosteroid drops—tension falls and facility of outflow increases to normal level usually within 2 months.
   - B. If tension remains elevated after 2 months, evaluate for an additional type of glaucoma.
   - C. Patient should have periodic examinations for development of open-angle glaucoma.
   - D. In conditions requiring steroids in spite of elevated tensions, epinephrine may be added.

Chandler, P. A. and Grant, W. M.: Lectures on Glaucoma. Philadelphia, Lea & Febiger, 1965, pp. 286-290.

Halasa, A. H.: The Basic Aspects of the Glaucomas. Springfield, Charles C Thomas, 1972, pp. 88-94.

RECESSED-ANGLE GLAUCOMA—elevation of the intraocular pressure following blunt trauma which gonioscopically demonstrates retroplacement of the lens-iris diaphragm and sectorally deepened anterior chamber with a tear in the anterior ciliary body

1. Characteristics
   - A. Onset of glaucoma is variable, within days up to years following trauma.
   - B. The severity of the glaucoma varies widely. Early onset of glaucoma may be related to the amount of angle recession.
   - C. By gonioscopy the attachment of the iris root appears farther posterior than normal. The scleral spur may stand out abnormally white, and the ciliary band may be widened. Recession may be in only one sector, multiple sectors, or even 360 degrees.
   - D. With onset of bilateral open-angle glaucoma, the eye with traumatic recession may be more difficult to control.
2. Treatment–The more extensive the angle damage, the less responsive to medical treatment.
   - A. Management same as that for open-angle glaucoma (see p. 60)
   - B. Observation for possible glaucoma for the remainder of patient's life if angle is recessed

Blanton, F. M.: Anterior Chamber Angle Recession and Secondary Glaucoma. Arch. Ophthal. 72:39-43, 1964.

Chandler, P. A. and Grant, W. M.: Lectures on Glaucoma. Philadelphia, Lea & Febiger, 1965, pp. 218-227.

Duke-Elder, S.: System of Ophthalmology, Vol. XI. St. Louis, C. V. Mosby, 1969, pp. 707-712.

Layden, W. E.: Traumatic Glaucoma. Trans. Amer. Acad. Ophthal. Otolaryng. 78:346-351, 1974.

Petit, T. H. and Keates, E. U.: Traumatic Cleavage of the Chamber Angle. Arch. Ophthal. 69:438-444, 1963.

Wolff, S. M. and Zimmerman, L. E.: Chronic Secondary Glaucoma: Associated with Retrodisplacement of Iris Root and Deepening of the Anterior Chamber Angle Secondary to Contusion. Amer. J. Ophthal. 54:547-562, 1962.

GLAUCOMA DUE TO ELEVATED EPISCLERAL VENOUS PRESSURE

1. Differential diagnosis—unusual except for direct arteriovenous communication. With dilated episcleral vessels rule out:
   A. Glaucoma, untreated
   B. Uveal neoplasm with localized engorgement
   C. Occlusion of orbital veins of the apex of the orbit
      (1) Endocrine exophthalmos of rapid development
      (2) Inflammatory lesions
      (3) Orbital thrombophlebitis
      (4) Neoplasm (rare)
      (5) Ligation
   D. Arteriovenous shunts including orbital, carotid-cavernous sinus and internal carotid-jugular vein
   E. Right-sided heart failure due to bronchitis, emphysema, bronchiectasis, or other type of chronic respiratory difficulty
   F. Increased viscosity of circulating blood
      (1) Polycythemia vera
      (2) Leukemia (early)
   G. Tetralogy of Fallot
   H. Obstruction of episcleral veins by caustic agents, radiation or trachoma
   I. Obstruction of vortex veins by inflammation, thrombosis or mechanical causes
   J. Obstruction of jugular veins by phlebitis
   K. Obstruction of superior vena cava by mediastinal tumor or ligation
2. Clinical characteristics
   A. Blood in Schlemm's canal (see p. 35)
   B. Congestion of episcleral and conjunctival vessels
   C. With arteriovenous communication, pulsating exophthalmos or bruit over affected side
   D. Neovascular glaucoma with fibrovascular membrane over the angle of the anterior chamber (see p. 34)
   E. Peripheral anterior synechiae
3. Treatment
   A. Surgical correction of the arteriovenous fistula

B. If surgery not feasible or unsuccessful, pressure controlled as an open-angle glaucoma (see p. 60)

C. With neovascular glaucoma, see treatment page 85.

Boniuk, M.: The Ocular Manifestations of Ophthalmic Vein and Aseptic Cavernous Sinus Thrombosis. Tran. Amer. Acad. Ophthal. Otolaryng. 76:1519-1534, 1972.

Chandler, P. A. and Grant, W. M.: Lectures on Glaucoma. Philadelphia, Lea & Febiger, 1965, pp. 274-275.

Duke-Elder, S.: Diseases of the Outer Eye. System of Ophthalmology, Vol. VIII, Part 1. St. Louis, C. V. Mosby, 1965, pp. 17-20.

Kolker, A. E. and Hetherington, J.: Becker-Shaffer's Diagnosis and Therapy of the Glaucomas, 3rd ed. St. Louis, C. V. Mosby, 1970, p. 257.

Minas, T. F., and Podos, S. M.: Familial Glaucoma Associated with Elevated Episcleral Venous Pressure. Arch. Ophthal. 80:202-213, 1968.

Podos, S. M., Minas, T. F., and Macri, F. J.: A New Instrument to Measure Episcleral Venous Pressure. Arch. Ophthal. 80:209-213, 1968.

Weekers, R. and Delmarcelle, Y.: Pathogenesis of Intraocular Hypertension in Cases of Arteriovenous Aneurysm. Arch. Ophthal. 48:338-343, 1952.

HEMOLYTIC GLAUCOMA—hyphema causing a secondary open-angle glaucoma

1. Differential diagnosis of hyphema
   A. Trauma
      (1) To iris, as iridodialysis
      (2) To ciliary body, as cyclodialysis
      (3) Tear of ciliary body—postcontusion deformity of anterior chamber
   B. Overdistension of vessels
      (1) Sudden lowering of high intraocular pressure
      (2) Obstruction of central retinal vein
   C. Fragility of vessel walls with iritis, as acute herpetic, gonorrheal or rheumatoid
   D. Blood derangement
      (1) Hemophilia

(2) Anemias
(3) Leukemia
(4) Purpura

E. Metabolic disease
(1) Scurvy
(2) Diabetes

F. Neovascularization of iris (see p. 34)

G. Vascularized tumors of iris
(1) Angioma
(2) Lymphosarcoma
(3) Juvenile xanthogranuloma–infant
(4) Retinoblastoma–infant

H. Persistent hyperplastic vitreous

I. Retrolental fibroplasia

J. Retinoschisis

2. Characteristics–commonly induced by trauma and associated with recurrent hyphemas filling most of the anterior chamber; blood staining of the cornea common

3. Treatment

A. Bed rest

B. Head elevated 30 degrees

C. Movement of pupil debatable as miotic or mydriatic

D. Binocular eye patches if desired

E. Elevated tension controlled with carbonic anhydrase inhibitors and osmotic agents. If uncontrolled, consider evacuation of blood from anterior chamber

F. Careful evaluation after hyphema clears for associated injuries to retina, chamber angle, lens, and optic nerve

Chandler, P. A. and Grant, W. M.: Lectures on Glaucoma. Philadelphia, Lea & Febiger, 1965, pp. 214-218.

Darr, J. L. and Passmore, J. W.: Management of Traumatic Hyphema. Amer. J. Ophthal. 63:134, 1967.

Duke-Elder, S. and Perkins, E. S.: Diseases of the Uveal Tract. System of Ophthalomology, Vol. IX. St. Louis, C. V. Mosby, 1966, pp. 19-20.

Edwards, W. E. and Layden, W. E.: Traumatic Hyphema. Amer. J. Ophthal. 75:110-116, 1973.

Gilbert, H. D. and Jensen, A. D.: Atropine in the Treatment of Traumatic Hyphema. Ann. Ophthal. 5:1297-1304, 1974.

Guzak, S. V.: Lymphoma as a Cause of Hyphema. Arch. Ophthal. 84:229-231, 1970.

Hogan, M. J. and Zimmerman, L. E.: Ophthalmic Pathology, 2nd ed. Philadelphia, W. B. Saunders, 1962, p. 145.

Howard, G. M.: Spontaneous Hyphema in Infancy and Childhood. Arch. Ophthal. 68:615-620, 1962.

Kwito, M. L. and Costenbader, F. D.: Glaucoma due to Secondary Hyphema. Amer. J. Ophthal. 53:590, 1962.

Rakusin, W.: Traumatic Hyphema. Amer. J. Ophthal. 74:284-292, 1972.

Roy, F. H.: Ocular Differential Diagnosis, 2nd ed. Philadelphia, Lea & Febiger, 1975, pp. 283-285.

Sears, M. L.: Surgical Management of Black-Ball Hyphema. Trans. Amer. Acad. Ophthal. Otolaryng. 74:820, 1970.

Yasuna, E.: Management of Traumatic Hyphema. Arch. Ophthal. 91: 190-191, 1974.

ANGLE-CLOSURE GLAUCOMA—increased intraocular pressure with closed angle demonstrated in gonioscopy

1. Characteristics–common in hyperopic, narrow chamber angle eyes which have small anterior segments. Tension elevation tends to occur abruptly causing typical symptoms of halos, hazy vision, and ocular pain. With pupillary resistance to the forward flow of aqueous and a laxity of the peripheral iris there is a forward displacement of the peripheral iris leading to closure of the anterior chamber angle.
2. Types
   A. Prodromal or intermittent angle closure–May have rapid increases and decreases of intraocular pressure. Symptoms may consist of foggy or hazy vision with rainbow-colored halos around lights. Ocular congestion, discomfort or headache may occur and then spontaneously go away within a few hours if the pupillary block is relieved. This may be precipitated by pupillary dilatation resulting from iatrogenic intervention, emotional upset or being in darkened area. Rare with miosis.
   B. Acute angle closure–Characteristics may include angle

closure by gonioscopy, blurred, foggy vision with colored halos around lights, pupil in a vertical oval mid-dilated fixed position, engorged iris and conjunctival blood vessels, mild aqueous flare, pain or discomfort, nausea and vomiting, generalized constriction of visual fields, hyperemic and edematous discs, anterior and/or posterior synechiae, localized iris atrophy and small anterior subcapsular lens changes.

C. Chronic angle closure–There is a gradual increase of the area of contact between the iris and the trabecular meshwork, usually starting at the upper angle and spreading inferiorly. There may be a progressive rise in pressure which may reach 40 to 60 mm Hg without discomfort, pain, halos, or congestion. The individual may have visual field defects very similar to those in open-angle glaucoma or chronic simple glaucoma. In some cases, peripheral anterior synechiae are formed.

3. Treatment–Medical therapy is used to normalize the intraocular pressure and consists of hyperosmotic agents. If it fails, surgical treatment is undertaken.

A. Osmotics
   (1) Oral glycerol, 50% solution, 1 cc/lb body weight
   (2) Urea, 1 to 1.5 gm/kg body weight
   (3) Mannitol, 20%, 1 to 2 gm/kg body weight
   With I.V., solutions given to a rate up to 60 drops/minute.

B. Miotics
   (1) 2% pilocarpine
   (2) Caracholin 1.5%
   (3) Eserine ointment 0.5%

   One drop instilled 3 times one minute apart, every 15 minutes for four hours.

C. Carbonic anhydrase inhibitors–Diamox 500 mg given by mouth and 250 mg repeated every four hours. If patient nauseated or vomiting, 500 mg Diamox dissolved in 10 cc sterile water with 250 mg I.M. and 250 mg I.V.

D. Retrobulbar anesthetic agents–1.5 ml of 2% Xylocaine or 2% procaine to decrease aqueous production and pain.

This is rarely used, for fear of a retrobulbar hemorrhage in an engorged eye and since hyperosmotic agents are available.

E. General measures
   (1) Morphine sulfate 50 mg s.c. or
   (2) Demerol 50 to 100 mg s.c.

F. Surgical therapy
   (1) Intensive medical therapy to normalize the intraocular pressure, then a few days for the eye to quiet before surgery
   (2) If the pressures cannot be normalized, posterior sclerotomy and vitreous aspiration and iridectomy
   (3) If the pressure can be normalized, peripheral iridectomy
   (4) Filtering operation reserved for peripheral iridectomy failures
   (5) Postoperative cycloplegics contraindicated with a narrow angle; miotics may be needed after iridectomy to maintain a normal intraocular pressure

G. Management of the fellow eye: While the acute glaucoma is being treated the fellow eye should be treated with pilocarpine solution to avoid angle closure. A prophylactic iridectomy should be done when the first eye is out of danger.

Bhargara, S. K., Leighton, D. A., and Phillips, C. I.: Early Angle Glaucoma: Distribution of Iridotrabecular Contact and Response to Pilocarpine. Arch. Ophthal. 89:369-372, 1973.

Chandler, P. A. and Grant, W. M.: Lectures on Glaucoma. Philadelphia, Lea & Febiger, 1965, pp. 157-192.

Foulds, W. S. and Phillips, C. I.: Some Observations on Chronic Closed-Angle Glaucoma. Brit. J. Ophthal. 41:208-213, 1957.

Friedman, Z. and Neumann, E.: Comparison of Prone-Position, Dark-Room, and Mydriatic Tests for Angle-Closure Glaucoma Before and After Peripheral Iridectomy. Amer. J. Ophthal. 74:24-27, 1972.

Gorin, G.: Re-evaluation of Gonioscopic Findings in Angle-Closure Glaucoma: Static versus Manipulative Gonioscopy. Amer. J. Ophthal. 71:894-897, 1971.

Harris, L. S. and Galin, M. A.: Prone Provocative Testing for Narrow Angle Glaucoma. Arch. Ophthal. 87:493-496, 1972.

Kessler, J.: A Discussion of the Mechanism of Chronic Angle-Closure Glaucoma. Amer. J. Ophthal. 46:888-890, 1958.

Kolker, A. E. and Hetherington, J.: Becker-Shaffer's Diagnosis and Therapy of the Glaucomas, 3rd ed. St. Louis, C. V. Mosby, 1970, pp. 175-205.

Lowe, R. F.: Primary Angle-Closure Glaucoma; Inheritance and Environment. Brit. J. Ophthal. 56:13-20, 1972.

Murphy, M. B. and Spaeth, G. L.: Iridectomy in Primary Angle-Closure Glaucoma. Arch. Ophthal. 91:114-122, 1974.

Phillips, C. I.: Aetiology of Angle-Closure Glaucoma. Brit. J. Ophthal. 56:248-253, 1972.

Pollack, I. P.: Chronic Angle-Closure Glaucoma: Diagnosis and Treatment in Patients with Angles that Appear Open. Arch. Ophthal. 85:676-689, 1971.

Sugar, H. S.: Cataract Formation and Refractive Changes after Surgery for Angle-Closure Glaucoma. Amer. J. Ophthal. 69:747-749, 1970.

Sugar, H. S.: Management of Angle-Closure Glaucoma. Ann. Ophthal. 6:517-525, 1974.

ANGLE-CLOSURE GLAUCOMA AFTER SCLERAL BUCKLING OPERATION FOR RETINAL DETACHMENT

1. Characteristics
   - A. There is elevation of intraocular pressure one or two days after scleral buckling operations for retinal detachment, with or without scleral implant.
   - B. Iris-lens diaphragm is pushed forward so that the anterior chamber is narrowed both axially and peripherally and angle closure occurs.
   - C. A choroidal detachment may be present.

2. Treatment
   - A. With early recognition, treatment is started promptly to avoid permanent changes, as sector atrophy of the iris, Glaukomflecken, permanent anterior synechiae, and damage to optic nerve head.
   - B. If performed early, glaucoma may be relieved by release of suprachoroidal fluid and a peripheral iridectomy.

Chandler, P. A. and Grant, W. M.: Lectures on Glaucoma. Philadelphia, Lea & Febiger, 1965, pp. 204-207.

Halasa, A. H.: The Basic Aspects of the Glaucomas. Springfield, Charles C Thomas, 1972, pp. 101, 103.

ANGLE-CLOSURE GLAUCOMA DUE TO MULTIPLE CYSTS OF IRIS AND CILIARY BODY—rare type of angle-closure glaucoma

1. Characteristics
   A. Rapid onset of symptoms
   B. Considerable variation in depth of chamber angle with some areas closed and other areas open
   C. After iridectomy, cysts of the ciliary body noted in the coloboma. May be heavily pigmented or clear. The iris cyst may be seen at or behind the pupillary border, more frequently after pupillary dilatation. Iris cysts are dark brown and may be mistaken for melanoma
   D. With multiple cysts of the iris and ciliary body, heavy deposition of pigment in the corneoscleral meshwork
2. Treatment
   A. Recognition–Irregular closure of angle does not often occur in primary acute angle-closure glaucoma. May be suspected but not proved until after iridectomy when the cysts are visible.
   B. May recur to cause repeated angle closure if the posterior wall of cyst is injured. Iris cysts should be punctured with a needle knife and only rarely recur. This will help deepen anterior chamber if peripheral anterior synechiae have not occurred.
   C. In most cases after iridectomy, the glaucoma will be controlled with or without medication. In rare cases a filtering procedure is necessary.

Abrahamson, I. A. and Jacobsen, L.: Iris Cyst. J. Pediat. Ophthal. 9: 177-178, 1972.

Becker, S. C.: Clinical Gonioscopy. St. Louis, C. V. Mosby, 1972, pp. 155-160.

Chandler, P. A. and Grant, W. M.: Lectures on Glaucoma. Philadelphia, Lea & Febiger, 1965, pp. 208-209.

Gaertner, J.: Fine Structure of Pars Plana Cysts. Amer. J. Ophthal. 73:971-984, 1972.

Roy, F. H. and Hanna, C.: Spontaneous Congenital Iris Cyst. Amer. J. Ophthal. 72:97-108, 1971.

PUPILLARY BLOCK GLAUCOMA FOLLOWING CATARACT EXTRACTION—increased intraocular pressure with shallow or flat anterior chamber following cataract extraction

1. Differential diagnosis
   - A. Wound leak
   - B. Postoperative iridocyclitis (see p. 88)
   - C. Posterior vitreous detachment associated with pooling or retrovitreal aqueous
   - D. Dense, impermeable anterior hyaloid membrane
   - E. Air pupillary block
   - F. Nonperforating iridectomy
   - G. Swollen lens material behind the iris (see p. 91)
   - H. Subchoroidal hemorrhage

2. Characteristics
   - A. Positive Seidel fluorescein test if wound leak
   - B. Aphakic pupillary block requiring intact hyaloid
   - C. Formation of peripheral anterior synechiae after a period of time

3. Treatment
   - A. Prevention—correct placement of sutures and correct surgical procedures
   - B. Binocular patching—pressure dressing
   - C. Maximum pupillary dilatation with short-acting cycloplegics—with time, miotics may be considered
   - D. Carbonic anhydrase inhibitors to help lower tension
   - E. Hyperosmotic agents or oral glycerin
   - F. Topical steroids

G. Subconjunctival injection at the limbus of 0.1 ml of 1% atropine, 4% cocaine and 1/1,000 epinephrine
H. Surgical tap of vitreous cavity behind ciliary body to fill anterior chamber with air, peripheral iridectomy, vitreous face incision
I. Later water ingestion to improve aqueous formation
J. Closure of leaking wound or conjunctival pedicle flap

Chandler, P. A. and Grant, W. M.: Lectures on Glaucoma. Philadelphia, Lea & Febiger, 1965, pp. 234-244.

Cotlier, E. and Herman, S.: Aphakic Flat Anterior Chamber: Treatment by Anterior Vitriotomy. Arch. Ophthal. 86:506-516, 1971.

Francois, J.: Aphakic Glaucoma. Ann. Ophthal. 6:429-442, 1974.

Jaffe, N. S.: The Vitreous in Clinical Ophthalmology. St. Louis, C. V. Mosby, 1969, p. 169.

Kolker, A. E. and Hetherington, J.: Becker-Shaffer's Diagnosis and Therapy of the Glaucomas, 3rd ed. St. Louis, C. V. Mosby, pp. 175-196.

Sell, D. B.: Management of the Flat Anterior Chamber After Cataract Surgery. Ann. Ophthal. 3:201-208, 1971.

Shaffer, R. N.: A Suggested Anatomic Classification to Define the Pupillary Block Glaucomas. Invest. Ophthal. 12:540-542, 1973.

Sugar, H. S.: Treatment of Hypotony Following Filtering Surgery for Glaucoma. Amer. J. Ophthal. 71:1023-1033, 1971.

Taylor, D. M.: Is the Flat Anterior Chamber Syndrome Necessary? Arch. Ophthal. 74:161, 1965.

Veirs, E. R. and Tate, C. B., Jr.: Adjunctive Surgical Techniques For Glaucoma. Ann. Ophthal. 3:196-200, 1971.

Weisel, J. and Swan, K. C.: Mydriatic Treatment of Shallow Chamber After Cataract Surgery. Arch. Ophthal. 58:126, 1957.

MALIGNANT GLAUCOMA (ciliary block glaucoma)—postoperative shallowing or flattening of the anterior chamber with elevation of intraocular pressure. The term "malignant" is used because it is resistant to therapy.

1. Characteristics
   A. May develop after an operation for angle-closure glau-

coma, in which part of the angle is closed at the time of operation with or without elevated tension.

B. May occur after iridectomy, filtering operation, and cyclodialysis.

C. May occur day after operation, or days, weeks or months later.

2. Treatment (difficult)

A. Mydriatic-cycloplegic–atropine 4% and phenylephrine 10% each 4 or 5 times daily. Therapy may be decreased to atropine 1% daily or every other day for an *indefinite* period of time. Condition may recur with discontinuation of drops.

B. The intraocular pressure may be lowered by hypertonic solution, either orally or intravenously, and a maximum dose of Diamox.

C. Glaucoma operations are unsuccessful.

D. Lens extraction either with vitreous loss or incision of the hyaloid face may help.

E. Perilenticular incision of the vitreous–sclerotomy with iridectomy and opening of the anterior and posterior hyaloid membrane, with the lens in place. Cataract and retinal detachment may be complications.

F. Fellow eye management–intensive mydriatic-cycloplegic therapy absorbed systemically may precipitate angle-closure glaucoma in the other eye.

(1) Open-angle, normal tension–observe or consider prophylactic peripheral iridectomy.

(2) Some of angle closed, tension elevated–normalize tension with vigorous medical means (see p. 75) and perform peripheral iridectomy.

(3) Angle closed, tension elevated at time of operation–malignant glaucoma may develop. Treat according to previous plans outlined for malignant glaucoma.

Chandler, P. A.: A New Operation for Malignant Glaucoma. Trans. Amer. Ophthal. Soc. 62:408-419, 1964.

Chandler, P. A. and Grant, W. M.: Mydriatic-Cycloplegic Treatment in Malignant Glaucoma. Arch. Ophthal. 68:353-359, 1962.

Chandler, P. A. and Grant, W. M.: Lectures on Glaucoma. Philadelphia, Lea & Febiger, 1965, pp. 197-203.

Levene, R.: A New Concept of Malignant Glaucoma. Arch. Ophthal. 87:497-506, 1972.

Rieser, J. C. and Schwartz, B.: Miotic-Induced Malignant Glaucoma. Arch. Ophthal. 87:706-712, 1972.

Shaffer, R. N.: The Role of Vitreous Detachment in Aphakic and Malignant Glaucoma. Trans. Amer. Acad. Ophthal. Otolaryng. 58: 217-228, 1954.

Simmons, R. J.: Malignant Glaucoma. Brit. J. Ophthal. 56:263-272, 1972.

Sugar, H. S.: Bilateral Aphakic Malignant Glaucoma. Arch. Ophthal. 87:347-351, 1972.

Weiss, D. I. and Shaffer, R. N.: Ciliary Block (Malignant) Glaucoma. Trans. Amer. Acad. Ophthal. Otolaryng. 76:450-461, 1972.

ESSENTIAL ATROPHY OF THE IRIS WITH GLAUCOMA

1. Characteristics
   A. Usually unilateral
   B. Women affected more frequently than men
   C. Distortion or displacement of the pupil in early or middle adult life but still reaction to light
   D. Peripheral anterior synechiae attached from the iris to the cornea at or anterior to Schwalbe's line
2. Types and treatment
   A. Progressive essential atrophy of the iris—There is progressive distortion of the pupil and disappearance of the stroma and then the pigment layer of the iris. Pupil may be distorted in several directions at once. Medical means to control glaucoma may be effective (see p. 64). When the peripheral anterior synechiae become extensive, surgical treatment may be necessary. Filtration surgery is most effective, but cyclodialysis and cyclodiathermy have been helpful in some cases. Filtration surgery is best performed in an area where the angle is open, and as much iris tissue as possible is removed from around the

filtering site. If surgery is performed at a late stage, the results are disappointing and often complicated, with loss of vitreous and obstruction of the filtering site with vitreous. Early extensive basal iridectomies might be of value.

B. Chandler's syndrome—Corneal edema secondary to corneal endothelial dystrophy is more pronounced than the iris atrophy. These patients primarily complain because of blurred vision and colored halos around lights in one eye. The goal of treatment is to keep the cornea clear by lowering the intraocular pressure. Early in the course of this disease, the tension may be lowered to normal and the corneal edema disappears, but later the edema may persist even when the tension is normalized. Optic nerve damage is rare. Medical therapy is the same as that for open-angle glaucoma (see p. 64). Operation as filtering surgery is indicated if the corneal edema is not controlled on maximum medical therapy.

Becker, S. C.: Clinical Gonioscopy. St. Louis, C. V. Mosby, 1972, pp. 136-139.

Chambers, J., et al.: Iris Atrophy in Sickle Cell Disease. Amer. J. Ophthal. 77:247-250, 1974.

Chandler, P. A.: Atrophy of the Stroma of the Iris: Endothelial Dystrophy, Corneal Edema and Glaucoma. Amer. J. Ophthal. 41: 607-615, 1956.

Chandler, P. A. and Grant, W. M.: Lectures on Glaucoma. Philadelphia, Lea & Febiger, 1965, pp. 276-285.

Cross, H. E. and Maumenee, A. E.: Progressive Spontaneous Dissolution of the Iris. Survey Ophthal. 18:186-199, 1973.

Jampol, L. M., Rosser, M. J., and Sears, M. L.: Unusual Aspects of Progressive Essential Iris Atrophy. Amer. J. Ophthal. 77:353-357, 1974.

NEOVASCULAR GLAUCOMA—growth of fibrovascular tissue over the surface of the iris (rubeosis iridis) and trabecular meshwork with impairment of aqueous outflow and elevation of intraocular pressure. Chamber angle neovascular tissue may lead to peripheral anterior synechiae

1. Characteristics
   - A. Onset of symptoms may be gradual or acute.
   - B. The intraocular pressure may be 80 to 90 mm Hg in severe cases.
   - C. History may reveal long-standing diabetes or a sudden or gradual loss of vision in the affected eye of 2 to 4 months' duration (occlusion of central retinal vein or artery).
   - D. Hyperemia of the globe, corneal epithelial edema and neovascularization of iris and chamber angle give the diagnosis in an acute elevation of pressure.
   - E. With a gradual onset of neovascular glaucoma, the cornea may be clear and the patient relatively asymptomatic in spite of IOPs from 40 to 50 mm Hg. Often a slight aqueous flare with a few cells may be noted.

2. Differential diagnosis of rubeosis iridis
   - A. Proximal vascular disease
     - (1) Aortic arch syndrome
     - (2) Carotid occlusive disease
     - (3) Carotid ligation
     - (4) Carotid cavernous fistula (see p. 72)
     - (5) Cranial arteritis
   - B. Ocular vascular disease
     - (1) Central retinal vein thrombosis–look for preexisting glaucoma; look at other eye
     - (2) Central retinal artery thrombosis–look for preexisting glaucoma; look at other eye
     - (3) Long posterior ciliary artery occlusion
   - C. Retinal diseases
     - (1) Diabetes mellitus–frequently associated with retinitis proliferans and recurrent vitreous hemorrhages
     - (2) Leber's miliary aneurysms

(3) Coats' disease
(4) Eales' disease
(5) Sickle-cell retinopathy
(6) Retinal hemangioma
(7) Persistent hyperplastic primary vitreous
(8) Retrolental fibroplasia
(9) Retinoblastoma
(10) Norrie's disease
(11) Retinal detachment
(12) Melanoma of choroid
(13) Glaucoma, chronic

D. Iris tumors
(1) Melanoma
(2) Metastatic carcinoma
(3) Hemangioma

E. Postinflammatory
(1) Uveitis, chronic
(2) Retinal detachment surgery
(3) Fungal endophthalmitis
(4) Radiation

F. Vascular tufts at the pupillary margin
(1) Myotonic dystrophy
(2) Cataract
(3) Diabetes mellitus
(4) Respiratory failure
(5) Ocular hypotonia

3. Treatment—Prognosis is guarded for vision; decision must be made as to goal: to make patient pain free or to save vision.

A. Occasionally if patient can tolerate the pain for about 6 weeks with pain medication, sedatives and reassurance, the eye frequently quiets down and the pain decreases even though the IOP remains high.

B. Medical therapy
(1) Miotics may aggravate symptoms and increase ocular congestion.
(2) Epinephrine and carbonic anhydrase inhibitors may be effective in lowering pressure.
(3) Mydriatic-cycloplegics as atropine or scopolamine

combined with glaucoma medication may help quiet eye.

(4) Steroids in frequent topical applications may help quiet eye. Periocular steroid injection may help decrease inflammation. Aristocort 1 cc of 40 mg/cc is injected with a 25-gauge needle through the lower lid periocular (Smith technique).

(5) Alcohol injection may be of value to decrease pain.

C. Surgical therapy

(1) Cryocyclotherapy for uncontrolled pain with use of narcotics and nonresponse to medications—2 applications per quadrant, total 8 lesions, starting 3 mm from limbus for 1 minute at —80 C with 2.5-mm retinal probe. Follow treatment with cycloplegics and steroids. If the pain is not controlled in 4 to 5 weeks repeat the cryocyclotherapy of 12 applications for 1 minute at —50 C rather than —80 C

(2) Enucleation—when other therapy is ineffective

Anderson, D. M., Morin, J. D., and Hunter, W. S.: Rubeosis Iridis. Canad. J. Ophthal. 6:183-188, 1971.

Bellows, A. R. and Grant, W. M.: Cyclocryotherapy in Advanced Inadequately Controlled Glaucoma. Amer. J. Ophthal. 75:679-684, 1973.

Boniuk, M.: Cryotherapy in Neovascular Glaucoma. Trans. Amer. Acad. Ophthal. Otolaryng. 78:337-343, 1974.

Bresnick, G. H. and Gay, A. J.: Rubeosis Iridis Associated with Branch Retinal Arteriolar Occlusions. Arch. Ophthal. 77:176-180, 1967.

Chandler, P. A. and Grant, W. M.: Lectures on Glaucoma. Philadelphia, Lea & Febiger, 1965, pp. 268-273.

Drews, R. C.: Steroid Management of Hemorrhagic Glaucoma. Trans. Amer. Acad. Ophthal. Otolaryng. 78:334-336, 1974.

Feibel, R. M. and Bigger, J. F.: Rubeosis Iridis and Neovascular Glaucoma. Evaluation of Cyclocryotherapy. Amer. J. Ophthal. 74:862-867, 1972.

Hoskins, H. D.: Neovascular Glaucoma: Current Concepts. Trans. Amer. Acad. Ophthal. Otolaryng. 78:330-333, 1974.

Kolker, A. E., and Hetherington, J.: Becker-Shaffer's Diagnosis and Therapy of the Glaucomas, 3rd ed. St. Louis, C. V. Mosby, 1970, pp. 241-242.

Madsen, P. H.: Rubeosis of the Iris and Haemmorrhagic Glaucoma in Patients with Proliferative Diabetic Retinopathy. Brit. J. Ophthal. 55:368-371, 1971.

Schulze, R. R.: Rubeosis Iridis. Amer. J. Ophthal. 63:487, 1967.

Wolter, J. R.: Double Embolism of the Central Retinal Artery and One Long Posterior Ciliary Artery Followed by Secondary Hemorrhagic Glaucoma. Amer. J. Ophthal. 73:651-657, 1972.

GLAUCOMA DUE TO INTRAOCULAR INFLAMMATION —signs and symptoms of inflammation may include cells, flare, keratitic precipitates, collections of inflammatory cells on the trabecular meshwork, anterior and/or posterior synechiae, or inflammatory foci in the peripheral fundus

1. Acute uveitis
   - A. Characteristics–hyperemia of the anterior segment, cells and flare, miosis, and keratitic precipitates. Usually the tension is *not* elevated. Must be differentiated from narrow-angle glaucoma which has less photophobia, a dilated pupil and narrowing of the chamber angle by gonioscopy.
   - B. Treatment–treatment of inflammation by topical administration of mydriatic-cycloplegic drugs as atropine and scopolamine and corticosteroids. Treatment of glaucoma with topical epinephrine and carbonic anhydrase inhibitors. Miotics are not usually used.
2. Herpetic keratitis and uveitis
   - A. Characteristics–dendritic staining pattern with inflammatory signs and symptoms. Inflammation may be so great that a hypopyon occurs.
   - B. Cytosine arabinocide or Stoxil ointment every hour helps diminish the corneal staining pattern. Cycloplegic-mydriatic drugs as atropine and scopolamine help decrease the inflammatory changes. Corticosteroids should not be used if the corneal changes are superficial. With deeper changes steroids can be used if the viral infection is also

controlled. Systemic carbonic anhydrase inhibitors are used to control the glaucoma.

3. Chorioretinitis
   A. Characteristics—inflammation of the posterior segment with evidence of inflammation of the anterior segment such as cells, flare, or keratitic precipitates
   B. Treatment—specific if etiologic agent found. Caution must be exercised in using corticosteroids because of corticosteroid-induced glaucoma (see p. 70). Treat glaucoma with epinephrine and carbonic anhydrase inhibitors.

4. Glaucomacyclitic crisis
   A. Characteristics—unilateral, recurrent attacks of glaucoma with cyclitic symptoms. Most common between ages of 20 to 50 years. Onset of symptoms is acute with minimal ocular discomfort, blurred vision, and colored halos around lights. The tension is usually 40 to 70 mm Hg with epithelial edema. The flare, cells and keratitic precipitates may take several days to develop and may be minimal.
   B. Treatment (glaucoma subsides in 1 to 3 weeks without treatment)—carbonic anhydrase inhibitors to control the elevated tension and steroids to control the inflammation. The inflammation recurs at intervals of a few months to a year or two. It stops at 50 to 60 years. Optic nerve damage and anterior and posterior synechiae seldom occur. The condition must not be confused with acute angle-closure glaucoma, which has a similar onset and symptoms.

5. Heterochromic iridocyclitis
   A. Characteristics—low-grade iridocyclitis, usually unilateral, with heterochromia and cataract. Peripheral anterior synechiae and posterior synechiae rarely develop. The glaucoma severity varies with glaucoma control. In some advanced cases, control may be difficult and field loss and cupping of the optic disc may occur. Gonioscopy may demonstrate fine new blood vessels in the chamber angle.

B. Treatment—inflammation usually not treated. The glaucoma is treated with miotics and carbonic anhydrase inhibitors. Filtering surgery may be of value to control the tension. Lens extraction does not alter the course of glaucoma. Since it is usually a unilateral disease, the eye can frequently be left in "reserve" and a lens extraction completed later. With medically uncontrolled tension following lens extraction, cyclodialysis is frequently done.

6. Sarcoid uveitis
   A. Characteristics—more frequent in Negro than Caucasian. The iris nodules may form localized synechiae with the keratitic precipitates to the trabecular meshwork. Posterior synechiae leading to iris bombé may occur. Small grayish vitreous balls may be seen in front of the retina.
   B. Treatment—initial good response to corticosteroids. Corticosteroids should be used with caution with extensive anterior synechiae.

7. Phacolytic glaucoma—inflammatory reaction secondary to degenerating lens protein
   A. Hypermature; lens in situ
      (1) Characteristics—unilateral glaucoma usually acute, but may be gradual with inflammatory reaction as flare, clumps of cells and keratitic precipitates (fine or mutton-fat). The chamber angle is open and a hypopyon may be present. Light perception with faulty projection may be present and does *not* indicate vision to be obtained postoperatively.
      (2) Treatment—removal of lens after lowering of tension medically. Corticosteroids may be used to decrease the inflammation postoperatively.
   B. Immature cataract; lens in situ
   Characteristics and treatment—difficult to establish diagnosis. If after the usual treatment for glaucoma secondary to uveitis (topical steroids, epinephrine, atropine, and carbonic anhydrase inhibitors) the uveitis and glaucoma gradually get worse, the lens should be removed. Many times the uveitis and glaucoma subside and the diagnosis is made in retrospect.

C. Completely dislocated cataract and glaucoma (rare)

(1) Characteristics—Cataract may be immature, mature or hypermature. The glaucoma is usually acute with a high pressure although onset may be gradual. The angle is open and there may be no other obvious cause for the glaucoma; thus the diagnosis is suspect. There may be a few cells in the aqueous and exudates on vitreous strands in the pupil.

(2) Treatment—If the pressure is high and not controlled by medical therapy, the lens should be removed. After a corneoscleral incision, an iridectomy and an inferior sphincterotomy are completed with gentle irrigation of the vitreous cavity, the lens floats up into the wound and can be removed. This is not always successful, however, so total vitrectomy with direct removal of the lens with cryo, forceps, or eresiphake has been used.

D. Phacolytic glaucoma due to retained lens cortex

(1) Characteristics—retained lens fragments following discission, perforating wound or extracapsular extraction. The eye may be inflamed, have keratitic precipitates, and/or cells or flare in the aqueous. Occasionally hypopyon is present and the angle is usually open unless peripheral anterior synechiae are present.

(2) Treatment

a. If little cortical material is present, atropine, corticosteroids and carbonic anhydrase inhibitors are used.

b. If much cortical material is present or the above treatment fails to control eyes with little cortical material, the residual lens cortex is removed by irrigation, forceps and scissors and possibly with the use of alpha-chymotrypsin.

E. Iris bombé

(1) Characteristics—active recurrent or chronic iritis or uveitis with inflammatory membrane which seals the iris to the lens; iris pushed forward by accumulation of aqueous in posterior chamber

(2) Treatment—peripheral iridectomy alone or with filtering procedure (if extensive peripheral anterior synechiae are present)

Chandler, P. A.: Completely Dislocated Hypermature Cataract and Glaucoma. Trans. Amer. Ophthal. Soc. 57:242-247, 1960.

Chandler, P. A.: Choice of Treatment in Dislocation of the Lens. Arch. Ophthal. 71:765-786, 1964.

Chandler, P. A. and Grant, W. M.: Lectures on Glaucoma. Philadelphia, Lea & Febiger, 1965, pp. 244-267.

Curran, R. E.: Surgical Management of Iris Bombé. Arch. Ophthal. 90:464-465, 1973.

Kass, M. A., Becker, B., and Kolker, A. E.: Glaucomacyclitic Crisis and Primary Open-Angle Glaucoma. Amer. J. Ophthal. 75:668-673, 1973.

Posner, A. and Schlossman, A.: Syndrome of Unilateral Recurrent Attacks of Glaucoma with Cyclitic Symptoms. Arch. Ophthal. 39: 517-535, 1948.

Posner, A. and Schlossman, A.: Syndrome of Unilateral Recurrent Attacks of Glaucoma with Cyclitic Symptoms. Trans. Amer. Acad. Ophthal. Otolaryng. 57:531-535, 1953.

Shaffer, R. N.: A Suggested Anatomic Classification to Define the Pupillary Block Glaucomas. Invest. Ophthal. 12:540-542, 1973.

Smith, R. E. and O'Connor, G. R.: Cataract Extraction in Fuchs' Syndrome. Arch. Ophthal. 91:39-41, 1974.

GLAUCOMA ASSOCIATED WITH DISLOCATION OF LENS

1. Differential diagnosis—Etiology varies, and may be traumatic, spontaneous and congenital. Try to identify etiology.
   A. Marfan's syndrome—usually superior displacement of lens
   B. Marchesani's syndrome—usually superior displacement of lens with spherophakia
   C. Dwarfism, genetic type
   D. Scleroderma
   E. Trauma as in Frenkel's syndrome (ocular contusion syndrome including recession of anterior chamber angle and surgical accidents (iatrogenic))
   F. Homocystinuria—usually downward displacement of lens

G. Syphilis
H. Spontaneous (degenerative)
I. Spherophakia
J. Autosomal recessive abnormality without other defects—usually ectopic pupils
K. Associated ocular findings
   (1) High myopia
   (2) Congenital glaucoma
   (3) Aniridia
   (4) Megalocornea
   (5) Coloboma of iris and choroid
L. Porphyria
M. Ehlers-Danlos syndrome
N. Rieger's syndrome
O. Hyperlysinemia
P. Sulfite oxidase deficiency

2. Characteristics and treatment—A subluxated lens is a displaced lens which remains in a plane behind the iris and within the patellar fossa. A luxated or dislocated lens is a lens displaced from the patellar fossa.
   A. Subluxation—displaced lens in patellar fossa. Consider pupillary block mechanism (p. 80), peripheral anterior synechiae (p. 33), or traumatic angle recession (p. 71) for cause of increased intraocular pressure. The cause of glaucoma indicates therapy, i.e., pupillary block indicates dilatation, other causes indicate miotics and carbonic anhydrase inhibitors. Rarely are peripheral iridectomies or filtering procedures necessary.
   B. Luxated lens—displaced lens removed from patellar fossa. In general, those lenses that can be trapped in the anterior chamber are surgically removed while those dislocated posteriorly are left alone except if secondary complications occur. Unfortunately one of these complications is glaucoma, which may force the clinician into surgical intervention where he would really prefer conservative management.

3. Types of glaucoma
   A. Pupillary block—Consider mydriatics and trap lens in anterior chamber prior to removal or, if lens has zonule

attachment and a formed vitreous face, attempt to trap behind the pupil. Then keep the pupil constricted with miotics or without a peripheral iridectomy. If a pupillary block is due to vitreous herniation, dilatation alone may suffice.

B. Peripheral anterior synechiae—Consider filtering procedure, cyclodialysis or cyclocryotherapy.

C. Phacolytic glaucoma—Treat medically with antiglaucoma medication and steroids and when eye is comparatively quiet remove the lens.

D. Post-traumatic recession—See page 71.

E. Acute glaucoma—See page 75. If lens is induced, remove it after eye is as quiet as possible.

F. Iridocyclytis—See page 88.

Chandler, P. A.: Completely Dislocated Hypermature Cataract and Glaucoma. Trans. Amer. Ophthal. Soc. 57:242-247, 1960.

Chandler, P. A. and Grant, W. M.: Lectures on Glaucoma. Philadelphia, Lea & Febiger, 1965, pp. 227-233 and 264-267.

Chandler, P. A.: Choice of Treatment in Dislocation of the Lens. Arch. Ophthal. 71:765-786, 1964.

Grant, W. M.: Open Angle Glaucoma Associated with Vitreous Filling the Anterior Chamber. Trans. Amer. Ophthal. Soc. 61:196-218, 1963.

Iliff, C. E. and Kramer, P.: A Working Guide for the Management of Dislocated Lenses. Ophthal. Surg. 2:251-257, 1971.

Jarrett, W. H.: Dislocation of the Lens. Arch. Ophthal. 78:289, 1967.

Jay, B.: Glaucoma Associated with Spontaneous Displacement of the Lens. Brit. J. Ophthal. 56:258-262, 1972.

Jensen, A. D. and Cross, H. E.: Surgical Treatment of Dislocated Lenses in the Marfan Syndrome and Homocystinuria. Trans. Amer. Acad. Ophthal. Otolaryng. 76:1491-1499, 1972.

Laster, L., et al.: A Previously Unrecognized Disorder of Metabolism of Sulfur-Containing Compounds: Abnormal Urinary Excretion of S-Sulfo-L-Cysteine, Sulfite and Thiosulfate in a Severely Retarded Child with Ectopia Lentis. J. Clin. Invest. 46:1082, 1967.

Rizzuti, A. B.: Complications in the Surgical Management of the Displaced Lens. Int. Ophthal. Clin. 5:3-54, 1965.

Smith, T. H., Holland, M. G., and Woody, N. C.: Ocular Abnormalities in Association with Hyperlysinemia. Trans. Amer. Acad. Ophthal. Otolaryng. 75:355-360, 1971.

Spaeth, G. D. and Barber, G. W.: Homocystinuria—Its Ocular Manifestations. J. Pediat. Ophthal. 3:42-48, 1966.

Strabismus Problems

Strabismus Problems

CONTENTS

Strabismus Problems

PRESENTING STRABISMUS PROBLEMS

1. Eye turning in, out or up
2. Closing one eye in bright sunlight or with higher visual demands
3. Decreased vision in one eye
4. Reading difficulties
5. Asthenopia—pulling of eyes or burning
6. Diplopia
7. Head position—head turn, head tilt and/or chin elevation or depression
8. Family history of strabismus
9. Routine examination picked up with tests such as cover-cover, cover-uncover, Polaroid stereopsis or 4△ test

STRABISMUS DATA BASE

1. History
   - A. Family history of strabismus
   - B. Pregnancy, labor, delivery and birth weight
   - C. Early and current development
   - D. General health (operations, hospitalizations, current medication, allergies)
   - E. Age of onset and duration
   - F. Course (intermittent or constant; progression)
   - G. Previous treatment

2. Examination
   A. Head position (head turn, head tilt and chin elevation or depression)
   B. Visual acuity (with and without correction, both distance and near)
      (1) Fixation pattern–central or eccentric, maintained or not maintained. If thought to be eccentric, visuoscope determines position as paramacular or parafoveal
      (2) Linear Snellen letters
      (3) Isolated E
   C. Binocular alignment–accommodative test target
      (1) Distance–primary, up, down, right, left and right and left head tilt. Exodeviation at greater than 20 feet
      (2) Near–primary
      (3) +3.00 lens–when ET greater near than distance and exotropia greater distance than near
      (4) Versions–weakness or overactions
      (5) Ductions–paralysis or restrictions
      (6) Tests
         a. Cover-uncover–tropia versus phoria
         b. Simultaneous prism-cover test
         c. Alternate cover–eso, exo, hyper
         d. Hirschberg
         e. Krimsky
         f. Near point of accommodation (N.P.C.)
   D. Sensory fusion
      (1) Worth 4-dot–fusion, suppression or diplopia (crossed or uncrossed)
      (2) Polaroid Stereo-Fly
      (3) Polaroid vectorgraph slides
      (4) Major amblyoscope
      (5) Scotoma plotting–strabismometer
   E. Motor fusion
      (1) Jampolsky 4△ test–unexplained decrease in monocular vision
      (2) Fusional vergence amplitudes D–6△; C–16△; D′–12△; C′–24△

(Cont'd p. 102)

STRABISMUS FLOW SHEET*

AGE		
DATE		
VISION	600	
OD = .	400	
OS = ×	300	
	200	
	100	
	70	
	50	
	40	
	30	
	20	
FUSION		
ESO DEV	60	
	45	
N = .		
	15	
D = X		
	0	
EXO DEV	15	
	30	
	45	
	60	

Rx
and
NOTES

* Reproduced with permission of Dr. Robert Reinecke, Professor of Ophthalmology, Albany Medical College, Albany, New York.

F. Retinal correspondence
   (1) Bagolini striated lens
   (2) Major amblyoscope
   (3) After-image

G. Cycloplegic refraction

H. Ophthalmoscopy

STRABISMUS TESTS

1. Alternate cover test (cover-cover test)
   A. Technique—fixate distant accommodative target
      (1) Cover one eye
      (2) Quickly move cover to other eye
      (3) Observe any movement of eye just uncovered
      (4) Repeat
   B. Interpretation—quantitative test to uncover total deviation (phoria and tropia) and direction of deviation (eso, exo, hyper)

2. Prism alternate cover test (prism cover-cover test)
   A. Technique—same as alternate cover test except prisms put before fixating eye and gradually increased until no movement with cover-cover test is found
   B. Interpretation—gives total amount of deviation

3. Cover-uncover test (monocular cover-uncover)
   A. Technique—fixate distant accommodative target
      (1) Cover right eye, observe the left eye for movement
      (2) Uncover right eye, observe both eyes for movement
      (3) Cover left eye, observe the right eye for movement
      (4) Uncover left eye, observe both eyes for movement
   B. Interpretation—qualitative test to determine direction (eso, exo, hyper) and nature (phoria or tropia) of deviation

4. Simultaneous prism-cover test
   A. Technique
      (1) Determine degree of tropia by cover-uncover test

(2) Place prism before deviating eye and at same moment cover before fixating eye

(3) If no movement correct prism strength

B. Interpretation—Amount of prism power is amount of tropia with superimposed phoria. Subtracting tropia found with cover-uncover test gives amount of phoria.

5. Hirschberg test (not precise)

A. Technique

(1) Fixation light is held 33 cm from patient

(2) Deviation of corneal light reflex from center of pupil is observed

B. Interpretation

(1) 1 mm decentration equals 7 degrees deviation (15△)

(2) Pupillary border decentration equals 15 degrees deviation (30△)

(3) Limbus decentration equals 45 degrees deviation (90△)

6. Krimsky test (not precise)

A. Technique

(1) Fixation light is held 33 cm from patient

(2) Prisms of increasing power are put before fixating eye until light reflex is centered in deviating eye

B. Interpretation—Amount of prism needed to center reflex in deviating eye gives estimate of ocular deviation.

7. Maddox rod test to determine heterophoria

A. Technique—horizontal deviation

(1) Maddox rod aligned horizontally before right eye

(2) Bright light presented at 20 feet (6M) in darkened room

B. Interpretation

(1) Vertical line through light—no horizontal phoria

(2) Vertical line to left of light—exophoria

(3) Vertical line to right of light—esophoria

8. Jampolsky 4△ prism test—detection of small-angle tropia

A. Technique—fixate distant accommodative target

(1) 4 △ base-out prism placed before right eye—both eyes observed for movement

(2) 4 △ base-out prism placed before left eye—both eyes observed for movement

(3) Above technique for small-angle esotropia. Base-in prism for small-angle exotropia

B. Interpretation

(1) Both eyes shift in direction of apex of prism, then eye without prism moves in opposite direction to recover —fusion

(2) Both eyes shift in direction of apex of prism but no recovery—monofixation with prism over fixating eye

(3) No shift of either eye—monofixation with prism over deviating eye

9. Worth 4-dot test

A. Technique

(1) Patient wears glasses with one red and one green lens

(2) Patient views fixation target of two green, one red and one white target

B. Interpretation—gross test of peripheral binocular cooperation only

(1) Four lights—normal fusion or ARC

(2) Two red or three green lights—suppression one eye

(3) Five lights—diplopia with uncrossed indicating esotropia or crossed indicating exotropia

10. Bagolini striated glass test

A. Technique

(1) Axis of striation oriented at 45 degrees right eye and 135 degrees left eye

(2) Fixation light at 33 cm and 20 feet (6M)

B. Interpretation

(1) Two lines completely going through light

a. Cover-uncover test reveals no shift and fixation is central—NRC

b. Cover-uncover test reveals shift and fixation is central—harmonious ARC

c. Cover-uncover test reveals shift and fixation is eccentric—eccentric fixation with harmonious ARC

(2) One line going through light and break in other line at light—foveal suppression with peripheral fusion

a. Cover-uncover test no shift—NRC
b. Cover-uncover test shift—ARC
(3) One line going through light—suppression of one eye
(4) Two lines each going through a light—NRC diplopia

11. Titmus or Wirt Stereo-Fly test
A. Technique (near test)—patient views test wearing Polaroid glasses
B. Interpretation
(1) Unable to see 3-D Stereo-Fly—no gross stereopsis
(2) 3-D Stereo-Fly, all animals, and 1-6 of circles—gross fusion with peripheral fusion
(3) 3-D of circles 7-9—central fusion

12. Polaroid vectorgraph slides
A. Technique (distant test)—patient views Polaroid vectorgraph slide with Polaroid glasses
B. Interpretation
(1) Patient reads across line—no scotoma
(2) Patient misses part of line—suppression scotoma

Bagolini, B. and Capobianco, N. M.: Subjective Space in Comitant Squint. Amer. J. Ophthal. 59:430-442, 1965.

Irvine, S.: A Simple Test for Binocular Fixation. Amer. J. Ophthal. 27:740-746, 1944.

Manley, D. R.: Symposium on Horizontal Ocular Deviations. St. Louis, C. V. Mosby, 1971, pp. 22-48.

Muenzler, W. S.: Combination Four-Dot Light. Amer. J. Ophthal. 69: 928, 1970.

Parks, M. M. and Eustis, A. T.: Monofixational Phoria. Amer. Orthopt. J. 11:38-45, 1961.

Pearlman, J. T.: Stereoscopic Vision Testing. Amer. Orthopt. J. 19: 78-86, 1969.

Raab, E. L.: Useful Extensions of Common Strabismus Tests: The Combined Worth 4-Dot Flashlight. Amer. Orthopt. J. 22:47-53, 1972.

Romano, P. E. and von Noorden, G. K.: Atypical Responses to the Four Diopter Prism Test. Amer. J. Ophthal. 67:935-940, 1969.

Scott, W. E. and Mash, J.: Steroacuity in Normal Individuals. Ann. Ophthal. 6:99-101, 1974.

von Noorden, G. K. and Maumenee, A. E.: Atlas of Strabismus. St. Louis, C. V. Mosby, 1973.

STRABISMUS THERAPEUTIC MODALITIES

Patching—patching one eye in relation to strabismus

1. Diagnostic
   - A. If symptoms are due to faulty binocular vision or muscle imbalance, patching the eye may decrease symptoms. For example, on an adult who has poorly compensated phoria with reading or watching TV, patch the eye for one week to see if the symptoms diminish.
   - B. For preoperative determination, for instance to determine between a divergence excess and a simulated divergence excess (basic exotropia), to rule out how much convergence tonus is present, patch the eye.
   - C. To bring out manifest deviation in a small child, patch one eye for 15 minutes, then observe.
   - D. To find out if sixth nerve palsy is a pseudoparalysis, use patching.
   - E. Patch the paretic eye in an ocular torticollis to determine if it is an ocular or a congenital torticollis (abnormality of the cervical vertebrae or sternocleidomastoid muscle).
2. Therapeutic
   - A. Paralytic strabismus to prevent diplopia
     - (1) Occlude the paretic eye to prevent diplopia.
     - (2) Occlude good eye to try to restore some movement to paralytic muscle.
     - (3) Use partial occlusion on the glasses if diplopia is in only one field of gaze.
   - B. Antiamblyopia treatment
     - (1) Patch the good eye constantly if central fixation is present.
     - (2) Avoid overpatching which might cause occlusion amblyopia. Patient age determines length of patching: for one year 7 to 10 days, for three years about 2 months, and for six years from 4 to 6 months. Return visits should be determined by patient age and fixation patterns should be checked on each visit to prevent occlusion amblyopia. Check patients under two years of age every 2 weeks.

C. Antisuppression in an alternating strabismus
   (1) Occlude the eyes alternately preoperatively: right eye one day, left eye next day.
   (2) Patching increases the foveal sensitivity, produces diplopia postoperatively, and holds progress made with orthoptics.

Miotics—parasympathomimetic drugs used to produce spasm of accommodation and a small pupil, as Phospholine iodide

1. Diagnostic (major value)
   A. Use with or without glasses to determine amount of accommodative esotropia.
   B. Postoperatively miotics may be used with a residual esotropia to determine if part of it is an accommodative esotropia and may be corrected with glasses.
   C. If the patient is wearing glasses and his condition is thought to be an undercorrected hyperopia, then miotics may be used. If a high AC/A ratio is present, i.e., esotropia at near decreases, a bifocal would be of value.
2. Treatment (limited value)
   A. Accommodative–for patient who does not tolerate glasses or for use in the summer for a few months
   B. With glasses–instead of bifocals with a high AC/A ratio or with bifocals with a high AC/A ratio which is not corrected with bifocals
   C. With a small or variable esotropia to hold fusion
   D. Postoperatively–undercorrection of esotropia or overcorrection of exotropia
   E. Medical patching–in patient who tolerates occlusive patching poorly. Miotics may be tried in amblyopic eye and atropine in eye with good vision. Most useful if a significant degree of hypermetropia is present, usually over 3 diopters
3. Undersirable side effects
   A. Systemic–nausea, abdominal cramps, diarrhea
   B. Ocular–iris cysts, anterior subcapsular cataract, pupillary block and angle closure, iritis and retinal detachment

4. Types of miotics used in strabismus
   A. Pilocarpine in 0.5 to 10%—duration of action 4 hours
   B. Echothiophate iodide in 0.06 to 0.25%—duration of action days to weeks
   C. Diisopropyl fluorophosphate in 0.035 to 0.1%—duration of action days to weeks

Cycloplegics—parasympatholytic drugs used to relax accommodation and dilate the pupil, as atropine

1. Refraction—to determine if the individual is hyperopic or myopic
2. Medical patching—if patient tolerates occlusive patching poorly. Atropine is used in the eye with the best vision and miotics in the amblyopic eye. Most useful if a significant degree of hypermetropia is present, usually over 3 diopters
3. To induce the patient to wear glasses—atropine for 3 to 4 weeks until the patient gets the habit of wearing his glasses
4. Accommodative spasm—to help the individual relax his accommodation so that his vision won't be blurred all the time
5. Undesirable side effects
   A. Systemic—hyperactivity to convulsions, hyperpyrexia, dry mouth
   B. Ocular—blurred vision
6. Types of cycloplegics used in strabismus
   A. Atropine, 0.5 to 2%—onset several hours, duration 2 weeks
   B. Homatropine, 1 to 5%—onset 1/2 to 1 1/2 hours, duration to 48 hours
   C. Cyclopentolate, 0.5 to 2%—onset 15 to 45 minutes, duration 24 hours
   D. Tropicamide, 1 to 2%—onset 20 to 25 minutes, duration about 6 hours

Glasses

1. Hyperopic individuals with accommodative esotropia—The full cycloplegic correction is given under four years of age. Over four years of age usually plus 1 is taken off the full

correction to be given, so the patient's vision will not be blurred.

2. With a high AC/A ratio with or without a deviation at distance but esotropia at near—A bifocal is of value. The full hyperopic correction is put on at distance and then approximately a plus 3 is given at near. The segment of the bifocals should be set up so that it splits pupil and the child will use it in reading position.
3. In myopia and exotropia—If the individual has a myopic correction overcorrection of myopic defect may decrease exotropia.
4. Astigmatism, myopia and hyperopia—Errors of significance must be corrected to get the best visual image to each macula. Only then can good visual acuity be obtained by eliminating suppression in amblyopia. The patient's age, visual requirements and mental capacity will help make this clinical determination.

Prisms

1. Diagnostic
   - A. Measure the deviation with the Krimsky method (light reflex), prism cover-cover method or simultaneous prism-cover test with a distant and near fixation target, to determine the deviation, including A and V syndromes and hypertropias
   - B. Measure the deviation in all fields of gaze to find whether the deviation is comitant or noncomitant
   - C. Measure amplitudes of fusions—break and recovery point of amplitude of convergence and amplitude of divergence.
   - D. Use clip-on prisms or Fresnel prisms to find if the symptoms are due to the deviation as a diagnostic trial.
2. Therapeutic
   - A. Induce diplopia as orthoptic exercise.
   - B. Build up fusional reserves in phorias.
   - C. Diminish the angle of squint in tropias by obtaining fusion with the angle and then decreasing the amount of prism.

D. Use Fresnel prisms, clip-ons, or prisms in glasses to overcome diplopia or decrease symptoms in phorias.
E. Use Fresnel prisms to produce fusion preoperatively.

3. Proper prescription of a prism
   A. Split the prism power between the two eyes.
   B. Six diopters per eye in conventional prism and 15 diopters in Fresnel prism are usually maximum.
   C. For functional position prescribe straight ahead or looking down in reading position.
   D. If the chin is elevated or depressed, prisms may overcome this problem if strabismus related.
   E. Prismatic effect
      (1) Grind into the lens
      (2) Fresnel paste-on plastic prisms
      (3) Clip-on prisms
      (4) Decentration, for instance with a plus 3 diopter sphere displaced inward 1 cm (10 mm) equals 3 diopters of base-in prism

Orthoptics—the examination and treatment of disturbances of binocular vision, excluding medical, optical and surgical treatment

1. Diagnostic
   A. Determination of fusion preoperatively to help determine whether surgery is cosmetic or functional (goal determination)
   B. Determination of fusion postoperatively to find if desired goal has been achieved (cosmetic or functional)
2. Therapeutic
   A. Almost constant good results with orthoptics alone
      (1) Convergence insufficiency
      (2) Horizontal heterophoria with functional signs
         a. Disturbed binocular vision as decreased amplitude of fusion or "diplopia" occurs
         b. Latent deviation must not be excessive
         c. Heterophoria persists but symptoms are gone after treatment
         d. Exophoria responds better than esophoria

(3) No help with vertical or torsional heterophoria
(4) Pure accommodative esotropia–Attempt to diminish the amount of plus needed or to get rid of glasses by use of exercise to strengthen fusion and amplitudes when child is old enough
(5) Some cases of intermittent exotropia
a. Small deviation that orthoptics alone will help
b. Surgery needed in addition
c. Alternate eye patching of value in intermittent exotropia

B. Almost constant good results with surgery and orthoptics
(1) Heterophoria–static deviation too large to be overcome by fusion alone
(2) Intermittent exotropia–surgery if deviation is too great or occurs too frequently
(3) Partial accommodative esotropia – surgery indicated on a nonaccommodative portion but orthoptics before and after surgery helpful for accommodative portion

3. Preconditions for orthoptics
A. Correct the amblyopia by patching (occlusive or medical).
B. Correct refractive and accommodative abnormalities with glasses prior to orthoptic treatment.

4. Contraindications
A. Age limit–varies around 6 but the best time for orthoptics is 4 to 8 years of age
B. When reeducation would lead to constant diplopia
C. Accurate age of onset of strabismus–congenital gives poorer response than later onset

ESOTROPIA—DIAGNOSTIC DECISIONS (may have more than one esotropia problem)

1. Esotropia varies in different fields of gaze
A. Vertical
(1) Greater up gaze than down gaze–A esotropia (p. 132)

(Cont'd p. 113)

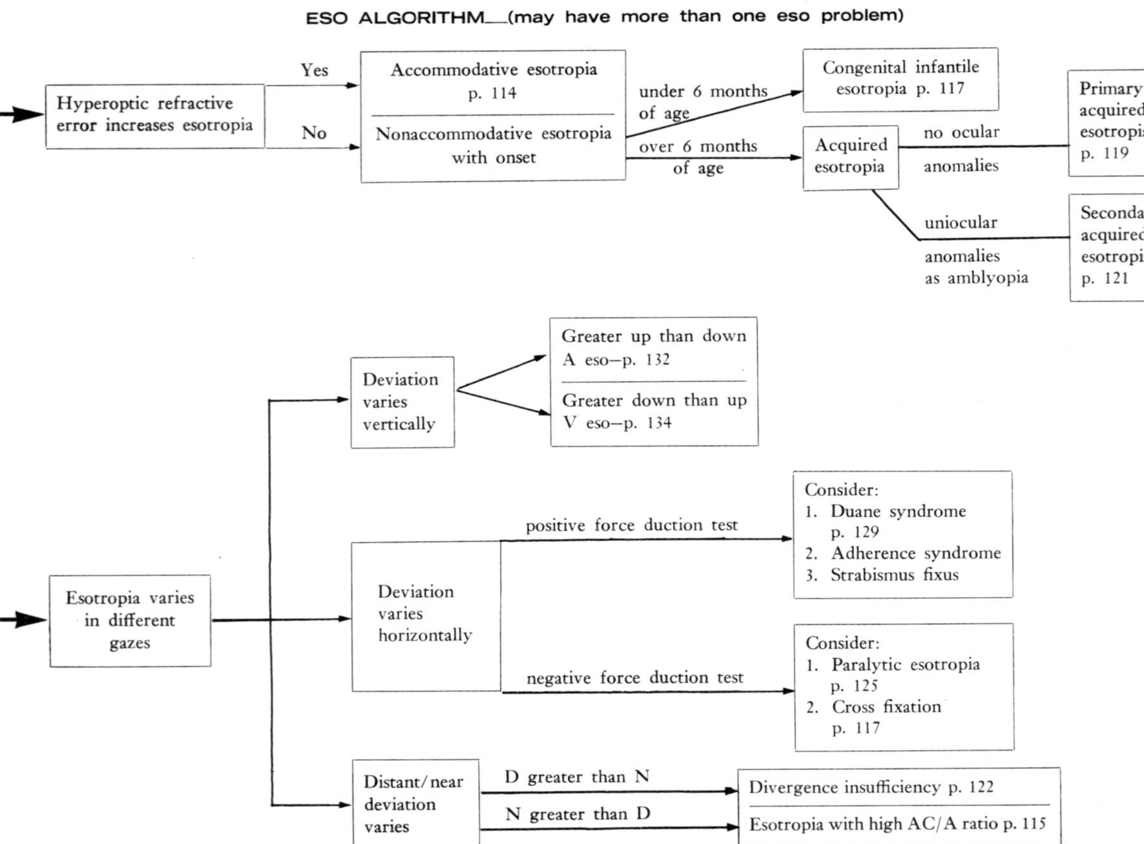
ESO ALGORITHM—(may have more than one eso problem)
Hyperoptic refractive error increases esotropia
Yes
No
Accommodative esotropia p. 114
Nonaccommodative esotropia with onset
under 6 months of age
over 6 months of age
Congenital infantile esotropia p. 117
Acquired esotropia
no ocular anomalies
uniocular anomalies as amblyopia
Primary acquired esotropia p. 119
Secondary acquired esotropia p. 121
Esotropia varies in different gazes
Deviation varies vertically
Greater up than down A eso—p. 132
Greater down than up V eso—p. 134
Deviation varies horizontally
positive force duction test
negative force duction test
Consider: 1. Duane syndrome p. 129 2. Adherence syndrome 3. Strabismus fixus
Consider: 1. Paralytic esotropia p. 125 2. Cross fixation p. 117
Distant/near deviation varies
D greater than N
N greater than D
Divergence insufficiency p. 122
Esotropia with high AC/A ratio p. 115

(2) Greater down gaze than up gaze–V esotropia (p. 134)

B. Horizontal
(1) Positive force duction test
a. Duane syndrome (p. 129)
b. Adherence syndrome
c. Strabismus fixus
(2) Negative force duction test
a. Paralytic esotropia (p. 125)
b. Cross fixation (p. 117)

C. Distance/near
(1) Distance greater than near–divergence insufficiency (p. 122)
(2) Near greater than distant–esotropia with high AC/A ratio (p. 115) (convergence excess)

2. Hyperopic refractive error increases esotropia
A. Yes–accommodative esotropia (p. 114)
B. No–nonaccommodative esotropia
(1) Onset under 6 months of age–congenital, infantile esotropia (p. 117)
(2) Onset over 6 months–acquired esotropia
a. No ocular anomalies–primary acquired esotropia (p. 119)
b. Uniocular anomalies as amblyopia, optic atrophy, or cataract–secondary acquired esotropia (p. 121)

PSEUDOESOTROPIA—an ocular appearance of esotropia when no manifest deviation of the visual axis is present

1. Prominent epicanthal fold
2. Negative angle kappa – pupillary light reflex displaced temporally
3. Telecanthus–the orbits normally placed, but the medial canthi far apart secondary to lateral displacement of the soft tissues
4. Abnormal shape of skull or thickness of skin surrounding the orbits

5. Lateral displacement of the concavity of the upper eyelid margin from the center of the pupil
6. Hypotelorism with narrow interpupillary distance
7. Entropion
8. Enophthalmos

Aita, J. A.: Congenital Facial Anomalies with Neurologic Defects. Springfield, Charles C Thomas, 1969.

Roy, F. H.: Ocular Differential Diagnosis, 2nd ed. Philadelphia, Lea & Febiger, 1975, p. 100.

Shaterian, E. T. and Weissman, I. L.: An Unusual Case of Pseudostrabismus. Amer. Orthopt. J. 23:68-70, 1973.

Urist, M. J.: Pseudostrabismus Caused by Abnormal Configuration of the Upper Eyelid Margins. Amer. J. Ophthal. 75:455-456, 1973.

von Noorden, G. K. and Maumenee, A. E.: Atlas of Strabismus, 2nd ed. St. Louis, C. V. Mosby, 1972, pp. 29-36.

ACCOMMODATIVE ESOTROPIA—convergent deviation associated with excess activation of accommodative convergence reflex

1. Clinical characteristics
   A. Accommodative esophoria–symptomatic asthenopia or diplopia after prolonged near work
   B. Accommodative esotropia
      (1) Onset between 1 to 7 years, most common at 2 years
      (2) Intermittent or constant
      (3) Frequent positive family history
      (4) Earlier the onset, worse the prognosis
   C. Findings–normal AC/A ratio tending to be associated with large hypermetropia (average + 4.75 sphere), high AC/A ratio more often seen with small hypermetropia (average + 2.25 sphere)
      (1) Sensory complications–suppression, amblyopia, or abnormal retinal correspondence

(2) Motor complications—hypertrophied medial recti producing nonaccommodative esotropia component superimposed upon the original accommodative esotropia
(3) May also have nonaccommodative or A or V esotropia

D. High AC/A ratio if near measurement is greater by 15△ or more than distance eso measurement with an accommodative target

2. Management
A. Under four years of age
(1) Full cycloplegic refraction for glass correction
(2) As a diagnostic trial in indeterminate cases, in children under 15 months of age or those with a high AC/A ratio, or as temporary therapy in children who will not accept glasses, 0.06% to 0.125% echothiophate (Phospholine iodide), isoflurophate (Floropryl) 0.025% ointment, or demecarium bromide (Humorsol) 0.125% or 0.25% daily. Daily instillation for 3 to 4 weeks, then one dosage every other day; gradually decrease to weekly instillation
(3) Bifocals with add of + 2.00 to + 3.00 if eyes are ortho at distance with correction but esotropic at near (high AC/A ratio). Bifocals must have high segment (split the pupil) to ensure use of adds for near seeing activities. Atropine 0.5% to 1% daily may be necessary initially to force use of the bifocals
(4) Occlusion therapy if amblyopia is present
(5) Surgery on that portion of esotropia that is not corrected by glasses, and surgery on significant associated problems such as overactions of inferior obliques, A-V syndromes, or high AC/A ratio
(6) Ocular examination every 6 months for well-controlled patients
a. Hypermetropia will usually be greater during the first five years of life
b. Abnormal AC/A ratio will usually improve regardless of treatment after age 8

B. Treatment 4 to 8 years of age
(1) Prescribe the minimum power lenses that provide

straight eyes at distance and near with adequate visual acuity. Usually it is necessary to take + 1.00 to + 1.50 from the cycloplegic refraction to prevent blurring of vision and patient resistance to glasses.

(2) Examine at 6-month intervals while under control.

(3) Conditions for bifocals, occlusion and surgery are the same as those described for children under 4 years.

(4) Orthoptics should be considered for combination of accommodative–nonaccommodative esotropia to eliminate suppression.

C. Treatment over age 8

(1) Some improve spontaneously as the hypermetropia decreases. The abnormal AC/A ratio tends to normalize and fusional divergence expands.

(2) Decrease or stop glasses if refraction is suitable.

a. Teach the patient to maintain straight eyes in the unaccommodative state without glasses, thus accepting blurred vision. Then small amounts of accommodation are allowed which are associated with increasing amounts of esophoria. Gradually the fusional divergence amplitude is built up so that larger exodeviations are withstood, until eventually clear vision and straight eyes are maintained. Physiological diplopia (framing) and bar reading during this routine help prevent suppression and esotropia from developing again. With time gradually stronger base-in prisms are employed while watching TV or reading to help increase the fusional divergence amplitude.

b. Diminish strength of miotics, i.e., gradually decrease Phospholine iodide to twice or once a week.

c. Use combination of orthoptics and weaker miotics.

d. Weaken glasses if vision is blurred or patient is exo with present lens. May decrease strength + 0.75 to 1.50 D at each time.

Abraham, S. V.: The Pre-operative and Post-operative Treatment of Strabismus with Miotics. J. Int. Coll. Surg. 40:375-379, 1963.

Breinin, G. M.: Accommodative Strabismus and the AC/A Ratio. Amer. J. Ophthal. 71:303-311, 1971.

Crawford, J. S. and Lewis, L.: The Diagnosis and Management of Accommodative Convergent Strabismus. Canad. J. Ophthal. 2:107-114, 1967.

Knapp, P.: The Clinical Management of Accommodative Esotropia. Amer. Orthopt. J. 17:8-13, 1967.

Manley, D. R.: Symposium on Horizontal Ocular Deviations. St. Louis, C. V. Mosby, 1971, pp. 49-71.

Ogle, K.: The Accommodative Convergence–Accommodation Ratio and Its Relation to the Correction of Refractive Error. Trans. Amer. Acad. Ophthal. Otolaryng. 70:322-330, 1966.

Rosenbaum, A. L., Jampolsky, A., and Scott, A. B.: Bimedial Recession in High AC/A Ratio. Arch. Ophthal. 91:251-253, 1974.

Sears, M. and Guber, D.: The Change in the Stimulus AC/A Ratio After Surgery. Amer. J. Ophthal. 64:872-876, 1967.

NONACCOMMODATIVE ESOTROPIA — convergent alignment of the visual axis not corrected by eliminating the accommodation convergence reflex

Congenital Infantile Esotropia — present prior to 6 months of age

1. Clinical characteristics
   - A. Large deviation (50 prism diopters or greater)
   - B. Usually good visual acuity in each eye; however, amblyopia may be present
   - C. Cross fixation (weakness of abduction and pseudopalsy of lateral rectus muscle) frequently present
     - (1) Vestibular stimulation–spin infant and look for ocular abduction
     - (2) Doll's head phenomenon–sudden passive turning of head may reveal good abduction in uncooperative child
     - (3) Diagnostic patching–patch nondeviating eye so that ocular movement of other eye can be noted
   - D. Frequently positive family history
   - E. Usually normal AC/A ratio

F. Frequently insignificant refractive error which does not influence esotropia (frequently hyperopic)
G. Untreated, absence of binocular function
H. Frequently overaction of inferior oblique muscles
I. May appear in neurologically abnormal infants, especially those with cerebral palsy
J. Abnormal musculature, abnormal attachments of tendons, or abnormal check ligaments which will be suspected with a positive forced duction test
K. Dissociated hypertropia in which double hyperphoria is present with cover-cover test

2. Management
   A. Occlusion therapy to prevent amblyopia, suppression and abnormal retinal correspondence, then alternate occlusion until time of surgery, to control fixation pattern
   B. Glasses—correct between 12 and 15 months of age
   C. Surgery if the infant is neurologically normal and the fixation is equal in both eyes. Esotropia may improve spontaneously with cerebral palsy or even become exotrophic with age
   D. Primary surgical procedure
      (1) Maximum bilateral medial rectus recession (4.5-5.5 mm) and removal of any fascial bands
      (2) Maximum medial rectus recession and lateral rectus recession (see p. 122 for amount)
      (3) Inferior oblique weakening procedure if needed
   E. With residual esotropia of 10 diopters or greater persisting six weeks after surgery, try Phospholine iodide to detect element of accommodative esotropia. Additional surgery may consist of:
      (1) Lateral rectus resection if previous bimedial rectus recession (see p. 120 for amount)
      (2) Medial rectus recession and lateral rectus resection if previous unilateral recession-resection (see p. 120 for amount)
   F. Prognosis for fusion potential good if the eyes ortho by two years of age, visual acuity equal in each eye, no associated eye problems, and the child neurologically normal

G. Surgery on older children (over 5 years)—usually cosmetic improvement but no fusion. Good cosmetic result is 15 to 20 diopters esotropia as eyes tend to diverge with age

H. Surgical correction of other associated strabismus problems as overaction of inferior oblique, A or V syndromes, etc.

I. May develop accommodative esotropia. With a residual postoperative esotropia, Phospholine iodide may be used to determine if an accommodative element is present. If present, hyperopic lens will be of value

Primary Acquired Esotropia—appears after 6 months of age with no ocular anomalies

1. Clinical characteristics
   - A. Smaller deviation than congenital esotropia
   - B. Amblyopia or alternate fixation
   - C. Small hypermetropic refractive error
   - D. Greater eso distance than near

2. Management
   - A. Occlusion therapy until maximum improvement in visual acuity is attained in the amblyopic eye, then alternate occlusion until the time of surgery
   - B. Accommodative element of esotropia (p. 114) treated by glasses or miotics
   - C. Orthoptics for fusion potential if the patient is four years of age or more and properly motivated. This helps define goal for surgery, i.e., cosmesis or fusion
   - D. Surgery
     - (1) Perform as soon as visual acuity in the amblyopic eye has reached maximum improvement, and after determining the nonaccommodative component, i.e., prism-cover test, fixating at distant object through fully corrected hypermetropic glasses that have been worn at least one month.
     - (2) Esotropia may improve spontaneously with cerebral palsy or even become exotropic with age.

(3) Surgically correct nonaccommodative component when 15 diopters or more and cosmetically noticeable.

a. Symmetrical surgery (after forced duction test)—Recess each medial rectus muscle 1 mm for each 10 diopters of deviation plus 0.5 mm for contraction of tissue due to suturing, to a maximum of 4.5 mm for patients 14 years old or younger and 5.5 mm for those older than 14 years.

Examples:

20 diopters—recess each MR 2.5 mm
30 diopters—recess each MR 3.5 mm
40 diopters—recess each MR 4.5 mm
50 diopters—recess each MR 4.5 mm and resect 1 mm of one lateral rectus muscle for each 5 of deviation starting at 4 mm for 50 diopters
60 diopters—recess each MR 4.5 mm and resect 6 mm of one LR. Additional surgery is performed in the event residual esotropia of 10 diopters persists six weeks following the initial surgery by resecting the lateral recti (see divergence insufficiency p. 122 for amount)

b. Asymmetrical surgery (after forced duction test)—Recess the medial rectus muscle and resect the lateral rectus muscle according to the amount of deviation present. The nonfixating eye is usually the eye operated upon. For esotropia of 20 △ or more, recess one medial rectus 4.5 mm (maximum) for patients up to age 14 years and 5.5 mm (maximum) for patients older than 14 years and resect one lateral rectus 1 mm/5 △ of deviation, starting at 4 mm for 20 △. The recession is maximum in each instance; only the resection varies and 10 mm is usually the upper limit.

Example (patients less than 14 years old):

20 △—recess MR 4.5 mm and resect LR 4 mm
30 △—recess MR 4.5 mm and resect LR 6 mm
40 △—recess MR 4.5 mm and resect LR 8 mm
50 △—recess MR 4.5 mm and resect LR 10 mm

For more than 50 △—recess both MR 4.5 mm and resection LR 4 mm or more as deviation increases

Additional surgery is performed in the event residual esotropia of 10 △ persists six weeks following the initial surgery, by recession of the medial rectus muscle and/or resection of the lateral rectus muscle. May not want to weaken inferior oblique muscle at same time.

(4) Prognosis is good for a binocular result if the eyes are straight while wearing glasses, visual acuity is equal in both eyes and there are no associated eye problems. The potential for fusion is shown with Bagolini striated lens.

(5) Surgically correct any other coexisting strabismus problems as overaction of inferior obliques or A or V esotropia.

Secondary Acquired Esotropia—appears after 6 months of age with uniocular anomaly

1. Clinical characteristics
   - A. Unilateral anomaly as unimproved amblyopia or sensory impairment in one eye including high myopia, unilateral cataract or unilateral optic atrophy
   - B. Anisometropia impairing the vision in one eye
2. Management
   - A. Glasses with the full cycloplegic correction in order to determine nonaccommodative component of the esotropia
   - B. Orthoptics usually not of value, but occlusion therapy may be
   - C. Surgery—undercorrection of surgically nonaccommodative component of esotropia since the amblyopic eye will gradually diverge with time. Surgery on the amblyopic eye usually consists of a recession of the medial rectus and resection of the lateral rectus
     - (1) ET of 20 △ or more—see page 120
     - (2) ET less than 20 △ which the surgeon feels must be corrected—recession of one MR 4.5 mm (for patients

age 14 or younger) and resection of the ipsilateral LR 4 mm. A single MR recession is usually ineffective

D. Adult patients with large-angle amblyopic esotropia
   (1) Forced abduction with forceps with dimpling or indentation sign, medial conjunctional recession 5 to 6 mm
   (2) Recession of medial rectus of amblyopic eye 5 to 6 mm
   (3) Resection of lateral rectus 12 to 14 mm (large resection results in limited adduction, but prevents recurrent esotropia)

Divergence Insufficiency

1. Characteristics—greater esodeviation far than near (low AC/A ratio), e.g., a patient may have an ET of 30 △ at distant and 10 △ at near. Sometimes associated with congenital myopia or following miotic treatment

2. Treatment
   A. Lateral rectus resection. Resect both LRs 1 mm/5 △ of deviation, starting at 4 mm for each eye for 20 △ of ET. This usually corrects the far error without overcorrecting the near

      Examples:

      20 △ ET at distance—resect both LRs 4 mm
      30 △ ET at distance—resect both LRs 6 mm
      40 △ ET at distance—resect both LRs 8 mm
      50 △ ET and over—resect both LRs 8 mm and recess one medial rectus (MR) 2.5 mm for each 5 prism diopters of deviation plus 0.5 mm for loss of tissue due to suturing
      60 △—resect each LR 8 mm and recess one MR 3.5 mm

   B. Recess medial rectus and resect lateral rectus—see page 120

Divergence Paralysis—supranuclear etiology with comitant esotropia of sudden onset and uncrossed diplopia at distance, fusion at near (usually 1 to 2 meters), normal ductions and versions, and gross impairment of fusional amplitudes of divergence

1. Differential diagnosis
   A. Epidemic encephalitis
   B. Syphilis
   C. Multiple sclerosis
   D. Head injuries
   E. Vascular disease
      (1) Occlusion of subclavian artery with flow reversal in vertebral artery
      (2) Hypertension
      (3) Vertebral basilar insufficiency
      (4) Diabetes mellitus
   F. Increased intracranial pressure
   G. Cerebral hemorrhage
   H. Diphtheria
   I. Poliomyelitis
   J. Influenza
   K. Lead poisoning
   L. Brain stem lesions
      (1) Hemangioma
      (2) Cerebellar cyst
      (3) Tumors as cerebellar and acoustic neuromas
   M. Functional
   N. Unknown

2. Characteristics
   A. Esotropia at distance
   B. Ortho at near
   C. Normal abduction

3. Treatment—surgery if condition persists and neurological status permits (see p. 122)

Burian, H. M. and Brown, A. W.: Unusual Adverse Effect of Prismatic Corrections in A Child with Divergence Insufficiency. Amer. J. Ophthal. 74:336-339, 1972.

Chamlin, M. and Davidoff, L.: Divergence Paralysis with Increased Intracranial Pressure. Arch. Ophthal. 46:145, 1951.

Cunningham, R. D.: Divergence Paralysis. Amer. J. Ophthal. 74:630-633, 1972.

Duke-Elder, S. and Scott, G. I.: System of Ophthalmology, Vol. XII. St. Louis, C. V. Mosby, 1971, pp. 833-835.

Dyer, J. A.: Atlas of Extraocular Muscle Surgery. Philadelphia, W. B. Saunders, 1970, pp. 143-147.

Dyer, J. A.: Some Pitfalls with Simultaneous Inferior Oblique Tenotomy (Disinsertion) and Lateral Rectus Resection. J. Pediat. Ophthal. 10: 47-53, 1973.

Fisher, N. F., Flom, M. C., and Jampolsky, A.: Early Surgery of Congenital Esotropia. Amer. J. Ophthal. 65:439-443, 1968.

Ing, M., et al.: Early Surgery for Congenital Esotropia. Amer. J. Ophthal. 61:1419-1427, 1966.

Lowe, B.: Orthoptic Treatment of Non-Accommodative Esotropia. Amer. Orthopt. J. 13:49-56, 1963.

Lyle, T. K.: A Review of the Results of Treatment of an Unselected Series of Cases of Non-Paralytic Convergent Strabismus in Children. Amer. Orthopt. J. 14:60-64, 1964.

Manley, D. R.: Symposium on Horizontal Ocular Deviations. St. Louis, C. V. Mosby, 1971, pp. 7-18.

Raskind, R. H. and Burian, H. M.: Bilateral Resections: Evaluation of Results of Bilateral Lateral Rectus Resections and Bilteral Medial Rectus Resections at the University of Iowa 1946-1966. Amer. J. Ophthal. 64:78-89, 1967.

Rutkowski, P. C. and Burian, H. M.; Divergence Paralysis Following Head Trauma. Amer. J. Ophthal. 73:660-662, 1972.

Taylor, D. M.: Congenital Strabismus: The Common Sense Approach. Arch. Ophthal. 77:478-484, 1967.

von Noorden, G. K., Isaza, M. E., and Parks, M. E.: Surgical Treatment of Congenital Esotropia. Trans. Amer. Acad. Ophthal. Otolaryng. 76:1465, 1972.

Walsh, F. B. and Hoyt, W. F.: Clinical Neuro-Ophthalmology, 3rd ed. Baltimore, Williams & Wilkins, 1969.

PARALYTIC ESOTROPIA (NONCOMITANT ESOTROPIA)—esotropia worse in lateral field of gaze of that paralytic lateral rectus. Greater esotropia when the paralytic eye fixes; thus the secondary deviation is greater than the primary deviation

1. Clinical features–Improvement is usually manifested three months after onset if it is to be forthcoming. Allow 6 to 12 months before assessing degree of recovery. Comitance tends to develop in unimproved cases due to contracture of direct antagonist, e.g., the medial rectus of the involved eye. Patient frequently will have face turn toward involved muscle to diminish diplopia, i.e., right face turn for right lateral rectus palsy. *Rule out CNS disease.*

2. Differential diagnosis of sixth nerve palsy
   A. Intracerebral
      (1) Thrombosis or aneurysm of nutrient vessels to sixth nucleus–basilar artery
      (2) Wernicke's encephalopathy–thiamine deficiency in alcoholics with sixth nerve palsy, paresis of horizontal conjugate gaze, nystagmus, ataxia, and Korsakoff's psychosis
      (3) Millard-Gubler syndrome–pontine lesion such as glioma with homolateral sixth nerve palsy, contralateral hemiplegia and homolateral peripheral facial palsy
      (4) Tumors–intracranial, pontine glioma, or metastatic tumor from breast, thyroid gland, or nasopharynx
      (5) Platybasia (cerebellomedullary malformation syndrome)
      (6) Nuclear aplasia
      (7) Foville's syndrome–homolateral sixth nerve palsy, homolateral peripheral facial palsy, homolateral horizontal gaze palsy, possibly combined with Horner's syndrome.
   B. Intracranial
      (1) Meningitis
      (2) Skull fractures
      (3) Carotid artery aneurysm
      (4) Gradenigo's syndrome–osteitis of petrous tip of

pyramid following homolateral mastoid or middle ear infection; facial pain (fifth nerve involvement)

(5) Subdural hematoma

(6) Increased intracranial pressure

(7) Cerebellopontine angle tumor, such as acoustic neuroma, producing unilateral deafness, facial paralysis, diplopia, and papilledema

(8) Neuritis due to diseases such as diabetes mellitus, herpes zoster, poliomyelitis, lead or arsenic poisoning, multiple sclerosis, syphilis, brucellosis

(9) Congenital absence of sixth nerve

(10) Myasthenia gravis

C. Lesions affecting exit of sixth nerve from the cranial cavity

(1) Cavernous sinus syndrome–paralysis of third, fourth and sixth nerves with proptosis

a. Cavernous sinus thrombosis

b. Pituitary adenoma, lateral extension

c. Aneurysm

d. Carotid-cavernous fistula

e. Extension of nasopharyngeal tumor

f. Extension from lateral sinus thrombosis

(2) Superior orbital fissure syndrome–same as for cavernous sinus syndrome except exophthalmos is less likely to occur and optic nerve involvement and miotic pupil are more likely

a. Sphenoid sinus suppuration

b. Skull fractures or hemorrhage

c. Tumors such as sphenoid ridge meningioma, nasopharyngeal tumor, and metastatic carcinomas

(3) Sphenopalatine fossa lesion – loss of tearing and paresis of second division of fifth nerve, most frequently due to malignant tumor

(4) Orbital apex lesion

D. Other

(1) Duane's syndrome–lateral rectus muscle replaced by fibrous band with adduction; eye retracts into orbit (p. 129)

(2) Lumbar puncture, lumbar anesthesia, or Pantopaque injection for myelography

(3) Toxic substances such as arsenic, carbon tetrachloride,

dichloroacetylene, Dilantin, gold salts, isoniazid, nitrofurantoin, thalidomide, trichloroethylene, furaltadone (Altafur).

3. Acquired isolated sixth nerve paresis in children
   A. Tumors—may be present with history of trauma or symptoms of infectious process
      (1) Primary
         a. Gliomas such as astrocytomas, ependymomas, and medulloblastomas
         b. Other primary tumors including meningiomas, pinealomas, craniopharyngiomas, and hemangiomas
      (2) Metastatic lesions such as those from the nasopharynx, rhabdomyosarcomas, and neuroblastomas
   B. Trauma—usually severe crush injury
   C. Inflammatory lesions such as meningoencephalitis, Gradenigo's syndrome (including fifth nerve), cerebellitis, and abscess
   D. Vascular lesions such as congenital aneurysm and arteriovenous anomalies
   E. Other
      (1) Hydrocephalus
      (2) Pseudotumor cerebri
      (3) Leukemia
      (4) Gaucher's disease
      (5) Lateral ventricular cyst
      (6) Spontaneous subdural hematoma
      (7) Transient in newborns
   F. Differential diagnosis must include unwillingness to cooperate, cross fixation, lack of effort in a habitually adducted eye, fibrosis of medial rectus, overambitious resection of medial rectus, Duane's syndrome, and bilateral horizontal gaze palsy. These may be differentiated by:
      (1) Patch test—Patching a nondeviated eye and forcing the use of the involved eye will help to differentiate between a true and pseudoparalysis of the lateral rectus in some instances.
      (2) Doll's head phenomenon—Sudden passive turning of the head will frequently reveal good abduction in an uncooperative child.

(3) Vestibular stimulatory test—Spin around with child in arms and observe for ocular abduction.
(4) Forced duction test—This will determine tight tissue.

4. Management—Rule out CNS disease.
   A. Caution—On all congenital paralytic esotropias do a forced duction test to rule out fibrous bands around medial rectus.
   B. On acquired esotropia, wait 6 to 8 months for return of function.
   C. Jensen's procedure—Recess the medial rectus of the involved eye 6 to 7 mm and unite lateral rectus to superior rectus and inferior rectus with suture.
   D. Resect palsied lateral rectus if some abduction is present. A 4-0 silk traction suture is placed in the insertion of the medial rectus muscle, threaded underneath the conjunctiva, above and below the corneal limbus, pulled out through the lateral canthus and tied over a button. Suture is left for 6 to 8 days.
   E. Other procedures
      (1) Recess the antagonist MR maximally (5.5 mm) and transplant the entire SR and IR nearly 90 degrees to be attached just above and below the LR insertion. The lateral rectus is not operated on.
      (2) Hummelshiem operation—Recess the medial rectus antagonist maximally, resect the paralytic LR maximally (10 mm) and transplant the temporal one third to one half of the SR and IR to a point just behind the LR insertion. This seldom helps.

Bedrossian, E. H.: Traction Sutures in the Treatment of Paralytic Esotropia. In: Symposium on Horizontal Ocular Deviations, (Manley, D. R. Ed.). St. Louis, C. V. Mosby, 1971, pp. 107-110.

Cogan, D. G.: Neurology of the Ocular Muscles, 4th ed. Springfield, Charles C Thomas, 1969, pp. 77-83.

Dyer, J. A.: Atlas of Extraocular Muscle Surgery. Philadelphia, W. B. Saunders, 1970, p. 154.

Ernest, J. T. and Costenbader, F. D.: Lateral Rectus Muscle Palsy. Amer. J. Ophthal. 65:721-726, 1968.

Frueh, B. R. and Henderson, J. W.: Rectus Muscle Union in Sixth Nerve Paralysis. Arch. Ophthal. 85:191-196, 1971.

Harley, R. D.: Complete Tendon Transplantation for Ocular Muscle Paralysis. Ann. Ophthal. 3:459-463, 1971.

Huber, A.: Eye Symptoms in Brain Tumors. St. Louis, C. V. Mosby, 1971, pp. 38-41.

Jampel, R. S. B. and Titone, C.: Congenital Paradoxical Gustatory Lacrimal Reflex and Lateral Rectus Paralysis. Arch. Ophthal. 67: 123-126, 1962.

Jensen, C. D. F.: Rectus Muscle Union: A New Operation for Paralysis of the Rectus Muscles. Trans. Pacif. Coast Otoophthal. Soc. 45:359-387, 1964.

Lignell, K. W. and Davis, C. J.: Abducens Nerve Palsy and Optic Disc Hypoplasia in Cretinism. J. Pediat. Ophthal. 8:105-106, 1971.

Metz, H. S., Scott, A. B., O'Meara, D., and Stewart, H. L.: Ocular Saccades in Lateral Rectus Palsy. Arch. Ophthal. 84:453-460, 1970.

Reisner, S. H., et al.: Transient Lateral Rectus Muscle Paresis in the Newborn Infant. J. Pediat. 78:461-465, 1971.

Robertson, D. M., Hines, J. D., and Rucker, C. W.: Acquired Sixth Nerve Paresis in Children. Arch. Ophthal. 83:574-579, 1970.

Roy, F. H.: Ocular Differential Diagnosis, 2nd ed. Philadelphia, Lea & Febiger, 1975, pp. 139-141.

Rucker, C. W.: The Causes of Paralysis of the Third, Fourth and Sixth Cranial Nerves. Amer. J. Ophthal. 61:1293, 1966.

Schrader, E. C. and Schlezinger, N. S.: Neuro-ophthalmologic Evaluation of Abducens Nerve Paralysis. Arch. Ophthal. 63:84-91, 1960.

Smith, J. L. and Creighton, J.: Sixth Nerve Palsy Due to Furaltadone (Altafur). Arch. Ophthal. 65:61-62, 1961.

Uribe, L. E.: Muscle Transplantation in Ocular Paralysis. Amer. J. Ophthal. 65:600-607, 1968.

Urist, M. J.: Lateral Gaze Palsy in Diabetic Lateral Rectus Paralysis. Ann. Ophthal. 6:583-593, 1964.

Walsh, F. B. and Hoyt, W. F.: Clinical Neuro-Ophthalmology. Baltimore, Williams & Wilkins, 1969.

Weintraub, M. I. and Sananman, M. L.: Giant Intracavernous Aneurysm and Sixth Nerve Palsy. Canad. J. Ophthal. 6:223-226, 1971.

DUANE RETRACTION SYNDROME—mimics sixth nerve paralysis

1. Clinical characteristics
   A. Decreased or absent abduction–noncomitant esotropia worse in gaze to affected side

B. Narrowing of the fissure and retraction of the globe on adduction
C. Widening of the fissure on attempted abduction
D. Normal or slight decrease in abduction
E. Usually seen in otherwise normal patients, primarily females, usually left eye
F. Vision usually unaffected and patients asymptomatic
G. Esotropia in primary position probably due to contracture of direct antagonist
H. Compensatory face turn toward involved muscle in order to maintain binocularity
I. Positive traction test in horizontal plane

2. Classification
   A. Duane I, which has primarily a palsy of abduction
   B. Duane II, in which there is a palsy of adduction (atypical or reverse Duane's) exotropia, worse on adduction
   C. Duane III, in which there is a palsy of abduction and adduction
   D. Etiology may be cocontraction of horizontal recti or fibrosis of lateral rectus
3. Treatment–to improve primary and head position
   A. If binocular vision is present in the straight-ahead position or to the uninvolved side, do not operate.
   B. With esotropia in primary position, recess the medial rectus contractured direct antagonist to improve mild compensatory face turn. With severe compensatory face turn, maximum recession of MR and resection of the ipsilateral LR is needed (see nonaccommodative esotropia associated with unimproved amblyopia for suggested amount) (see p. 122).
   C. If the eye is divergent treat as exotropia with amblyopia (see p. 143).
   D. Hummelschiem operation is usually of little value.
   E. Myotomy of the overactive inferior oblique, if present, may be of cosmetic value.
   F. Resection of lateral rectus alone increases enophthalmos.
   G. Recession of lateral rectus a few millimeters may decrease enophthalmos.

Agrawal, T. P.: Duane's Retraction Syndrome. Brit. J. Ophthal. 51:208-209, 1967.

Cross, H. E. and Pfaffenbach, D. D.: Duane's Retraction Syndrome and Associated Congenital Malformations. Amer. J. Ophthal. 73:442-449, 1972.

Dyer, J. A.: Atlas of Extraocular Muscle Surgery. Philadelphia, W. B. Saunders, 1970, p. 15.

Gobin, M. H. and Bierlaagh, J.: The Surgical Management of the Duane Syndrome and Sixth Nerve Paralysis. Brit. Orthopt. J. 28: 32-41, 1971.

Holtz, S. J.: Congenital Ocular Anomalies Associated with Duane's Retraction Syndrome, the Nevus of Oto, and Axial Anisometropia. Amer. J. Ophthal. 77:729-731, 1974.

Nawrotzki, I.: A Typical Retraction Syndrome: A Case Report. J. Pediat. Ophthal. 4:32-34, 1967.

Pfaffenbach, D. D., Cross, H. E., and Kearns, T. P.: Congenital Anomalies in Duane's Retraction Syndrome. Arch. Ophthal. 88: 635-639, 1972.

Scott, A. B. and Wong, G. Y.: Duane's Syndrome. Arch. Ophthal. 87:140-142, 1972.

Sevel, D. and Kassar, B. S.: Bilateral Duane Syndrome. Arch. Ophthal. 91:492-494, 1974.

Smith, J. L., et al.: Acquired Retraction Syndrome After Sixth Nerve Palsy. Brit. J. Ophthal. 57:110-114, 1973.

SMALL-ANGLE ESOTROPIA (MICROTROPIA, FIXATION DISPARITY, MONOFIXATIONAL ESOPHORIA, ESO FLICK)—peripheral fusion with small deviation of one fovea. Suppression of nonfixating macula prevents diplopia

1. Characteristics
   - A. Monofixation—diagnosed by monocular cover-uncover test, 4 △ base-out test, or visuoscope
   - B. Tropia—diagnosed by monocular cover-uncover test (up to 6 prism diopters) which may increase by cover-cover test
   - C. Amblyopia—common but usually not severe. Most 20/60 or better in the deviated eye

D. Usually harmonious ARC demonstrated by Bagolini striated lens
E. Peripheral fusion frequent–demonstrated by Worth 4-dot test and major amblyoscope
F. Fusional vergences such as amplitudes of fusion–normal or diminished
G. Stereopsis–stereopsis poorer than 60 seconds of arc by Wirt stereo test
H. Suppression of fovea of deviating eye–demonstrated by binocular perimetry or Polaroid vectorgraph slide
I. No visual symptoms, cosmetically straight eyes and condition stationary

2. Management–No therapy is indicated for small deviation unless glasses are needed to prevent accommodative esotropia, poor vision or asthenopia. Occlusion is for the minimal amblyopia in a child under 8 years of age.

Chamberlain, W.: The Significance of Monofixation Syndrome. J. Pediat. Ophthal. 10:252-255, 1973.

Epstein, D. L. and Tredici, T. J.: Microtropia (Monofixation Syndrome) in Flying Personnel. Amer. J. Ophthal. 76:832-841, 1973.

Helveston, E. M. and von Noorden, G. K.: Microtropia: A Newly Defined Entity. Arch. Ophthal. 78:272-281, 1967.

Lang, J.: Microtropia. Arch. Ophthal. 81:758, 1969.

Manley, D. R.: Symposium on Horizontal Ocular Deviations. St. Louis, C. V. Mosby, 1971, pp. 18-48.

A ESOTROPIA—esotropia greater looking up by 15 prism diopters than looking down

1. Clinical features
   A. An overaction of the superior oblique muscles or underaction of the inferior oblique or inferior rectus muscles may be present. For example, a right inferior oblique muscle underaction would demonstrate a left hypertropia which was worse in left gaze than right gaze and was worse in left head tilt than right head tilt (see p. 159).

B. Fusion may be obtained by chin elevation.
C. A mongoloid (upward) slant of the lid fissures may be present.
D. There may also be accommodative, nonaccommodative or paralytic esotropia components.

2. Management
A. Usually no surgery is indicated when there is only small angle of esotropia in primary position or looking down.
B. With marked underaction of the inferior oblique muscles and an angle of strabismus in primary position and below of sufficient size to warrant surgery, a bilateral tenotomy of the superior oblique muscles is recommended in combination with or followed by horizontal surgery. Bilateral tenotomy of the superior obliques may correct about 20 △ to 35 △ of A esotropia pattern up, but may increase an esotropia deviation of 10△ to 15△ in the primary position. With a continued A pattern and hypertropia, 6 mm or more tucking of the inferior oblique muscle is usually indicated.
C. With normal action of the oblique muscles, horizontal surgery may be indicated, with upward displacement of the medial recti or downward displacement of the lateral recti. For example, a patient with 0 deviation on downward gaze, 20 △ esotropia in the primary position, and 35 △ esotropia on looking up might have 2.5 mm medial rectus recession with upward movement of each muscle one muscle width (see nonaccommodative esotropia, p. 120). Bilateral resection of the lateral rectus muscle with downward movement of tendon corrects more esodeviation in up gaze than in down gaze and is satisfactory for moderate degrees of A esotropia (p. 122). With a recess-resect, recess and raise the medial rectus and resect and lower the lateral rectus.
D. Temporal placement of each superior rectus muscle tendon one full muscle width may increase divergence on upward gaze.
E. Treat accommodative (p. 114), nonaccommodative (p. 117), and paralytic (p. 125) esotropia components.

Bedrossian, E. H.: Bilateral Superior Oblique Tenectomy for the A Pattern in Strabismus. Arch. Ophthal. 78:334-336, 1967.

Dyer, J. W.: Atlas of Extraocular Muscle Surgery. Philadelphia, W. B. Saunders, 1970, pp. 143-144.

Hardesty, H. H.: Superior Oblique Tenotomy. Arch. Ophthal. 88: 181-184, 1972.

Harley, R. D.: A and V Patterns in Horizontal Deviations. In: Symposium on Horizontal Ocular Deviations (Manley, D. R., Ed.). St. Louis, C. V. Mosby, 1971, pp. 188-203.

Helveston, E. M.: Atlas of Strabismus Surgery. St. Louis, C. V. Mosby, 1973.

Jampolsky, A.: A and V Syndrome. Strabismus. New Orleans Academy Symposium. St. Louis, C. V. Mosby, 1962, pp. 157-177.

Manley, D. R. and Hughes, R. M.: Surgical Management of A Pattern Esotropia. Ann. Ophthal. 3:1067-1078, 1971.

Urist, M. J.: Recession and Upward Displacement of the Medial Rectus Muscles in A Pattern Esotropia. Amer. J. Ophthal. 65:769-773, 1968.

V ESOTROPIA—esotropia greater looking down by 15 prism diopters than looking up

1. Clinical features
   - A. Frequently, an underaction of the superior oblique or an overaction of the inferior oblique is present. For example, a right superior oblique underaction would demonstrate a right hypertropia which was worse in left gaze than right gaze and worse in right head tilt than left head tilt (see p. 158).
   - B. Antimongoloid (downward) slant of the lid fissures is frequent.
   - C. Fusion may be obtained by chin depression.
   - D. There may also be accommodative, nonaccommodative, or paralytic esotropia components.
2. Management
   - A. With an underaction of the superior oblique muscles, myotomy, tenotomy or recession of the inferior oblique muscles in combination with or followed by horizontal surgery is indicated. If the hypertropia is less than 10 $\triangle$

in adduction, no oblique surgery is needed. However, if the hypertropia is over 10 △ in adduction, a weakening procedure of the IO is indicated. Myotomy of the inferior oblique muscle may give up to 30 △ esotropia correction down, combined myectomy inferior oblique and tuck superior oblique give 45 △ esotropia correction down. With a continued V pattern and hypertropia, a tuck of 6 mm or more of superior oblique muscle may be the next procedure of choice.

B. When there is normal action of the superior oblique muscles, horizontal surgery alone as recession of both medial recti muscles with downward transplantation of their insertions is indicated (see nonaccommodative esotropia, p. 120). For example, if a patient has 0 deviation on upward gaze, 20 △ esotropia in primary position, and 40 △ esotropia on downward gaze, recession 2.5 mm medial rectus bilateral with downward displacement of each muscle one muscle width is indicated. When there is orthophoria in primary position and a small esotropia in downward gaze, temporal transplantation of the inferior rectus muscles one muscle width is recommended. With a recess-resect, recess and lower the medial rectus and resect and raise the lateral rectus.

C. Correct by conjugate-oblique prisms, prisms acting in same direction combined with prisms acting disjunctively —for example, OD 10 △ base down and 8 △ base out, OS 10 △ base down and 8 △ base out.

D. Treat accommodative (p. 114), nonaccommodative (p. 117), and paralytic (p. 125) esotropia components.

Diamond, S. V.: Esotropia Aided by Conjugate-Oblique Prism Correction: Case Report. Amer. J. Ophthal. 69:133-135, 1970.

Dyer, J. A.: Atlas of Extraocular Muscle Surgery. Philadelphia, W. B. Saunders, 1970, p. 144.

Dyer, J. A.: Some Pitfalls with Simultaneous Inferior Oblique Tenotomy (Disinsertion) and Lateral Rectus Resection. J. Pediat. Ophthal. 10:47-53, 1973.

Harley, R. D.: A and V Patterns in Horizontal Deviations. In: Symposium on Horizontal Ocular Deviations (Manley, D. R., Ed.). St. Louis, C. V. Mosby, 1971, pp. 188-203.

Stager, D. R. and Parks, M. M.: Inferior Oblique Weakening Procedures: Effect on Primary Position Horizontal Alignment. Arch. Ophthal. 90:15-16, 1973.

Urist, M. J.: A Technique for Recession of the Inferior Oblique Muscle. Arch. Ophthal. 87:198-201, 1972.

von Noorden, G. K. and Maumenee, A. E.: Atlas of Strabismus. St. Louis, C. V. Mosby, 1973, pp. 152-157.

EXOTROPIA—DIAGNOSTIC DECISIONS (may have more than one exotropia problem)

1. Fusion ability
   A. Fusion-exophoria (p. 138)
   B. Intermittent fusion–see #2
   C. No fusion–see #2
2. Exotropia varies in different fields of gaze
   A. Vertical
      (1) Greater up gaze than down gaze–V exotropia (p. 146)
      (2) Greater down gaze than up gaze–A exotropia (p. 144)
   B. Horizontal
      (1) With nystagmus consider internuclear ophthalmoplegia (p. 150)
      (2) With no nystagmus consider third nerve or medial rectus palsy (p. 147)
   C. Distant/near
      (1) Equal distant and near–basic exotropia (p. 141)
      (2) Near greater than distant–convergence insufficiency (p. 141)
      (3) Distant greater than near with + 3.00 lens, near exotropia increases
         a. No–divergence excess (p. 142)
         b. Yes–pseudodivergence excess (p. 142)

EXO ALGORITHM—(may have more than one exo problem)

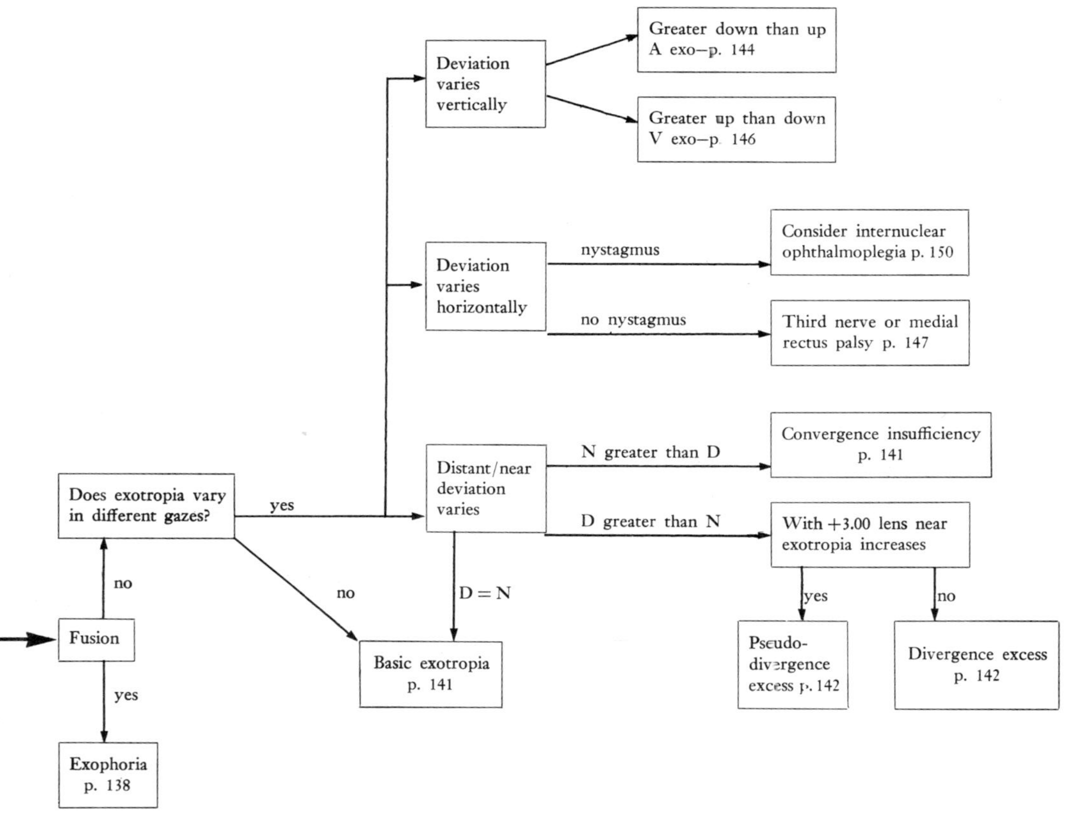

PSEUDOEXOTROPIA—an ocular appearance of exotropia when no manifest deviation of the visual axis is present

1. Hypertelorism with wide interpupillary distance
2. Positive angle kappa–pupillary light reflex displaced nasally
3. Exophthalmos
4. Narrow lateral canthus
5. Wide palpebral fissure
6. Displaced macula which may be the result of retrolental fibroplasia
7. Heterochromia when the lighter-colored eye appears to diverge

Lyle, T. K. and Wybar, K. C.: Lyle and Jackson's Practical Orthoptics in the Treatment of Squint. Springfield, Charles C Thomas, 1967, pp. 335-336.

Shaterian, E. T. and Weissman, I. L.: An Unusual Case of Pseudostrabismus. Amer. Orthopt. J. 23:68-70, 1973.

Roy, F. H.: Ocular Differential Diagnosis, 2nd ed. Philadelphia, Lea & Febiger, 1975, p. 102.

von Noorden, G. K. and Maumenee, A. E.: Atlas of Strabismus, 2nd ed. St. Louis, C. V. Mosby, 1972, pp. 29-36.

EXOPHORIA—divergent alignment held latent by the fusional and accommodative convergence reflexes. Diagnosed by cover-uncover test and alternate cover test

1. Clinical characteristics
   A. The condition is usually asymptomatic.
   B. If symptomatic, the following gradually develop: asthenopia, momentary diplopia and momentary blurred vision. These symptoms usually develop late in day or when ill or tired.
   C. Determine the AC/A ratio in exodeviation by measuring distant and near fixation. If there is a normal ratio the

distant and near exodeviation are similar (basic exophoria). If there is a low AC/A ratio, there is less convergence at near than distance, causing a greater exodeviation at near than distance (convergence insufficiency). If there is a high AC/A ratio, there is more convergence at near than distance, causing a greater exodeviation at distance than at near (divergence excess).

2. Management
   A. Absence of symptoms—no treatment
   B. With the presence of symptoms
      (1) Orthoptics build larger fusional convergence amplitude to compensate for exodeviation. Treatment is emphasized for distance if exo is greater at distance than near and near if exo is greater at near by using the following methods: major amblyopscope, physiological diplopia, loose prisms, stereoscope or orthofusor, bar reading, Polaroid television screen. Alternate eye patching may be of value.
      (2) Glasses can employ accommodative convergence to compensate for exodeviation by undercorrecting hypermetropia and overcorrecting the myopia. Compensating for the exodeviation by providing base-in prism power for spectacle is seldom done.
      (3) Surgery is indicated only if the exodeviation is large in distant fixation and symptoms are significant.

Abraham, S. V.: Exodeviations: I. Are Phorias Precursors to Strabismus? J. Pediat. Ophthal. 6:131-135, 1969.

Abraham, S. V.: Exodeviations: II. The Convergence Function and Its Relation to Phorias. J. Pediat. Ophthal. 6:213-219, 1969.

Abraham, S. V.: Exodeviations: III. Treatment of Exophoria. J. Pediat. Ophthal. 7:20, 1970.

Burian, H. M.: Exodeviations: Their Classification, Diagnosis and Treatment. Amer. J. Ophthal. 62:1161-1166, 1966.

Manley, D. R.: Classification of Exodeviations. In: Symposium on Horizontal Ocular Deviations (Manley, D. R., Ed.). St. Louis, C. V. Mosby, 1971, pp. 123-129.

EXOTROPIA—outward ocular deviation. May be constant or intermittent (latent deviation to manifest deviation). Diagnosed by cover-uncover test and alternate cover test

1. Clinical characteristics
   A. Usually appearing after six months of age, the condition is aggravated by distant fixation, fatigue, illness, upon first wakening, visual inattention, and bright sunlight. Often one eye is closed or covered with the hand particularly when tired, watching TV, or in bright sunlight. With suppression of deviating eye, may be asymptomatic.
   B. Frequently it is hereditary.
   C. Younger children tend to have a high AC/A ratio and are less exo at near than distance.
   D. A and V syndromes and hypertropias may be present.
   E. Diplopia is difficult to elicit because of suppression when eyes are exotropic. There is usually no amblyopia.
   F. May be caused by inbalance of tonic convergence-divergence–an anomaly impairing the vision of one eye, abnormal musculature, tendons, osteology or check ligament.

2. Management
   A. Glasses if needed, overcorrect myopia, undercorrect hyperopia by 0.75 to 1.50 D
   B. Alternate patching either eye to help increase the foveal sensitivity. Alternate patching each eye 2 days for several weeks before surgery. Surgery may be performed at a young age in order to prevent deepening of suppression, prevent possible deterioration to constant exotropia, and keep patient from annoying functional and cosmetic defect while young
   C. Treatment for amblyopia if present
   D. Orthoptics–occasionally used preoperatively for antisuppression and fusional convergence amplitude strengthening. Without surgery it is unusual for orthoptics to produce a life-long containment of the exodeviation. It can be tried as an adjunct to surgery if the patient is over four years of age and cooperative

E. Surgery with signs of exotropia progression

(1) Basic exotropia—see page 140 for characteristics and general management. The distance and near measurements are similar and thus the AC/A ratio is normal.

a. Symmetrical surgery—recess lateral rectus bilaterally to equator, about 6.5 mm for 15 years or younger and 7.5 mm for older patients

b. Asymmetrical surgery--preferred procedure if amblyopia is present. Recession of the LR of the exotropic eye to the equator, plus resection of the MR on same side as follows: resect a minimum of 4 mm for 20 △ diopters deviation and 1 mm more for each 5 diopters increase in XT to a maximum of 10 mm. With long-standing exotropia and dimpling of the conjunctiva on forced duction test on adduction, lateral conjunctival recession is valuable

Examples:

20 △ XT—recess LR to equator and resect MR 4 mm

30 △ XT—recess LR to equator and resect MR 6 mm

50 △ XT—recess LR to equator and resect MR 10 mm

More than 50 △ XT—recess LR to equator and resect MR 10 mm

(2) Convergence insufficiency exotropia—see page 140 for characteristics and general management. Greater exodeviation near than far, thus a low AC/A ratio. Symptomatic (asthenopia and diplopia) if not suppressed while doing near work.

a. Orthoptics to strengthen fusional convergence amplitude and correct refractive errors such as myopia, astigmatism, and balance anisometropia

b. Base-in prisms for near work of questionable value

c. Surgical treatment of no lasting value. Resect both MRs 4 mm/20 △ of XT and increase amount of resection of each muscle 1 mm/5 △ increase in XT

Examples:

20 △ XT–resect each MR 4 mm
30 △ XT–resect each MR 6 mm
40 △ XT–resect each MR 8 mm
50 △ XT or greater–recess LR to equator and resect MR 10 mm

(3) Divergence excess exotropia–see page 140 for characteristics and general management. Greater exodeviation for distance than near, thus a high AC/A ratio. + 3.00 lens does not change the near deviation. If far exodeviation constitutes a frank tropia or if it is intermittently greater than 20 △, operation may be advisable. The procedure of choice is bilateral LR recession to the equator, 6.5 mm for 14 years old or younger and 7.5 mm for older patients. In younger children with exotropia needing a bilateral LR recession, less than 20 △ 4 to 4.5 mm bilateral LR recession.

Examples:

20-25 △ XT–5 mm bilateral LR recession
24-35 △ XT–6 mm bilateral LR recession
Over 35 △ XT–7 mm bilateral LR recession
Less than 20 △–best not to operate. Alternating patching procedure of choice

(4) Pseudodivergence excess–greater exodeviation for distance than near, thus a high AC/A ratio. + 3.00 lens or short-term occlusion increases the near exo until it may almost equal the distance exodeviation. Treat as basic exotropia (p. 141).

(5) Management of surgical overcorrection

a. Immediate (transient postoperative esotropia)–ideal immediate result which usually disappears in one to two weeks without treatment

b. Late persistent postoperative esotropia associated with inactive accommodation–either plus lens or miotics, alternate occlusion to prevent further converging. Orthoptics may be tried in children 4 years or older with the hope of teaching recognition of differences between homonymous and heteronymous diplopia, also to train patient not to converge while attempting to eliminate homonymous diplopia (convergence must be relaxed and fusional divergence applied). Patient may need to wear base-in prisms for a while to get this started. Build fusional divergence amplitude.

c. Reoperation—delay six months or more since in many persistent cases the esotropia eventually disappears. If the need for reoperation is eventually conceded, handle surgically as though it were a fresh case.

(6) Management of surgical undercorrection

a. Prisms, excessive minus lens, patching and orthoptics to correct. Initial two months most flexible time for improvement

b. Reoperation on opposite muscle—for instance, resect the medial recti bilaterally if maximum lateral rectus recessions were done primarily after several months

(7) Adult patients with large-angle amblyopic exotropia

a. Forced adduction with forceps with dimpling or indentation sign, plan conjunctival recession 6 to 7 mm

b. Recession of amblyopic eye lateral rectus 7 to 8 mm

c. Resection of amblyopic eye medial rectus 12 to 14 mm (large resection results in limited abduction, but prevents recurrent exotropia)

Burian, H. M.: Exodeviations: Their Classifications, Diagnosis and Treatment. Amer. J. Ophthal. 62:1161-1166, 1966.

Burian, H. M. and Franceschetti, A. T.: Evaluation of Diagnostic Methods for the Classification of Exodeviations. Trans. Amer. Ophthal. Soc. 68:56-71, 1970.

Dunlap, E. A. and Gaffney, R. B.: Surgical Management of Intermittent Exotropia. Amer. Orthopt. J. 13:20-33, 1963.

Dyer, J. A.: Atlas of Extraocular Muscle Surgery. Philadelphia, W. B. Saunders, 1970, pp. 148-150.

Hardesty, H. H.: Treatment of Over-Corrected Intermittent Exotropia. Amer. J. Ophthal. 66:80-86, 1968.

Hardesty, H. H.: Treatment of Under and Over-Corrected Intermittent Exotropia with Prism Glasses. Amer. Orthopt. J. 19:110-119, 1969.

Hiles, D. A., Davies, G. T., and Costenbader, F. D.: Long-Term Observations on Unoperated Intermittent Exotropia. Arch. Ophthal. 80:436-442, 1968.

Hiles, D. A.: Current Concepts in the Management of Re-operations upon the Extra-ocular Muscles. Ann. Ophthal. 5:1344-1351, 1973.

Manley, D. R.: Classification of Exodeviations. In: Symposium on Horizontal Ocular Deviations (Manley, D. R., Ed.). St. Louis, C. V. Mosby, 1971, pp. 128-139.

Raab, E. L. and Parks, M. M.: Recession of the Lateral Recti: Early and Late Post-Operative Alignments. Arch. Ophthal. 82:203-209, 1969.

Rayner, J. W., et al.: Management of Adult Patients with Large Angle Amblyopic Exotropia. Ann. Ophthal. 5:95-99, 1973.

von Noorden, G. K.: Divergence Excess and Stimulated Divergence Excess: Diagnosis and Surgical Management. Docum. Ophthal. 26: 719, 1969.

Walsh, F. I.: Orthoptic Treatment of Intermittent Exotropia. Amer. Orthopt. J. 16:73-79, 1963.

A EXOTROPIA—exotropia greater looking down by 15 prism diopters than looking up

1. Clinical characteristics
   - A. Mongoloid (upward) slant of the lid fissures
   - B. Alternating sursumduction and associated vertical divergence
   - C. An overaction of the superior oblique muscles or underaction of the inferior oblique or inferior rectus muscles. For example, a right inferior oblique muscle underaction would demonstrate a left hypertropia which is worse in left gaze than right gaze and is worse in left head tilt than right head tilt (see p. 159)
   - D. Fusion obtained by chin depression
2. Management
   - A. When the oblique muscles are normal, move both LRs down the width of one muscle and recess each to the equator if XT is 20 △ or greater in the primary position.

Move LRs down one muscle width only but recess 0.5 mm to allow for loss of tissue in suturing if XT is less than 20 △ in the primary position.

B. With a persistent A pattern after operation on lateral rectus muscles (with normal oblique action), each inferior rectus muscle (IR) may be moved nasally the width of one muscle to improve ability to converge on downward gaze.

C. With definite overaction of superior oblique muscles on versions (underaction of inferior oblique), if XT is 20 △ or greater in the primary position, do an intrasheath tenotomy of both SOs. Weakening procedures on the superior obliques, such as complete bilateral tenotomy of the superior oblique tendons and sheaths, result in approximately 45 to 50 △ decrease in exodeviation in down gaze and approximately 15 △ decrease in the primary position with little effect on up gaze. One must have 45 △ of A exotropia down with demonstrable overaction of superior obliques for this procedure to be indicated in children.

D. Treat basic exotropia (p. 141), divergence excess (p. 142), pseudodivergence excess (p. 142), and convergence insufficiency components (p. 141). With convergence insufficiency and no oblique dysfunction, the medial rectus muscles may be resected and moved upward 5 mm.

Bedrossian, E. H.: Bilateral Superior Oblique Tenectomy for A Pattern in Strabismus. Arch. Ophthal. 78:334-336, 1967.

Dyer, J. A.: Atlas of Extraocular Muscle Surgery. Philadelphia, W. B. Saunders, 1970, p. 149.

Hardesty, H. H.: Superior Oblique Tenotomy. Arch. Ophthal. 88: 181-184, 1972.

Harley, R. D. and Manley, D. R.: Bilateral Superior Oblique Tenectomy in A-Pattern Exotropia. Ann. Ophthal. 2:441-448, 1970.

Harley, R. D.: A and V Patterns in Horizontal Deviations. In: Symposium on Horizontal Ocular Deviations (Manley, D. R., Ed.). St. Louis, C. V. Mosby, 1971, pp. 188-203.

Helveston, E. M.: A-Exotropia, Alternating Sursumduction and Superior Oblique Over-action. Amer. J. Ophthal. 67:377-380, 1969.

Jampolsky, A.: A and V Syndromes. Strabismus. New Orleans Academy Symposium. St. Louis, C. V. Mosby, 1962, pp. 157-177.

V EXOTROPIA—exotropia greater looking up by 15 diopters than looking down

1. Clinical characteristics
   A. Underaction of the superior oblique or overaction of the inferior oblique muscles. With an underaction of the right superior oblique you would expect a right hypertropia which is worse in left gaze than right gaze and worse in right head tilt than left head tilt (see p. 158)
   B. Antimongoloid (downward) slant of the lid fissures
   C. Fusion obtained by chin elevation

2. Management
   A. With "normal" oblique action, move both LRs upward the width of one muscle and recess to the equator if XT in the primary position is 20 △ or greater. If XT is less than 20 △ in the primary position, move LRs upward but recess only 0.5 mm to allow for loss of tissue in suturing.
   B. With persistent V pattern after operation on lateral rectus muscles (with normal oblique action), displace SRs nasally the width of one muscle to improve ability to converge eyes.
   C. With definite inferior oblique overaction bilaterally (underaction of superior oblique), recess LRs to equator for XT of 20 △ or more in primary position; bilateral IO weakening may be done. If XT is less than 20 △ in primary position do IO weakening only. Myotomy of the inferior oblique muscle gives about 20 △ exotropia correction in the up position and 5 △ and 10 △ exoreduction in the primary position. Full tuck of superior oblique gives about 20 △ correction in up position and myectomy IO and tuck SO 45 △ correction of exo in up position.
   D. Correct with conjugate-oblique prisms, prisms acting in same direction combined with prisms acting disjunctively —for example, OD 10 △ base down and 8 △ base out, OS 10 △ base down and 8 △ base out.
   E. Treat basic esotropia (p. 141), divergence excess (p. 142), pseudodivergence excess (p. 142), and convergence insufficiency components (p. 141).

Billet, E. and Freedman, M.: Surgery of the Inferior Oblique Muscles in V Pattern Exotropia. Arch. Ophthal. 82:21-22, 1969.

Diamond, S.: Conjugate and Oblique Prisms Correction for Noncomitant Ocular Deviations. Amer. J. Ophthal. 58:89, 1964.

Dyer, J. A.: Atlas of Extraocular Muscle Surgery. Philadelphia, W. B. Saunders, 1970, pp. 149-150.

Harley, R. D.: A and V Patterns in Horizontal Deviations. In: Symposium on Horizontal Ocular Deviations (Manley, D. R., Ed.). St. Louis, C. V. Mosby, 1971, pp. 188-203.

Helveston, E. M.: Atlas of Strabismus Surgery. St. Louis, C. V. Mosby, 1973.

Parks, M. M.: A Study of the Weakening Surgical Procedures for Eliminating Overaction of the Inferior Oblique. Trans. Amer. Ophthal. Soc. 69:163-187, 1971.

Stager, D. R. and Parks, M. M.: Inferior Oblique Weakening Procedures: Effect on Primary Position Horizontal Alignment. Arch. Ophthal. 90:15-16, 1973.

PARALYTIC EXOTROPIA (third nerve paralysis)

1. Characteristics—complete or incomplete
   - A. Lid ptosis
   - B. Pupil—dilated (internal ophthalmoplegia)
   - C. EOM—paralysis of SR, MR, IO and IR
   - D. Eye abducted and depressed due to intact LR and SO
2. Differential diagnosis
   - A. Intracerebral
     - (1) Lesion of red nucleus (Benedikt's syndrome)—homolateral oculomotor paralysis with contralateral intention tremor
     - (2) Syndrome of cerebral peduncle (Weber's syndrome)—homolateral oculomotor paralysis and crossed hemiplegia
     - (3) Occlusion of basilar artery—due to emboli especially but also to hemorrhage or aneurysm
     - (4) Recurrent third nerve palsy secondary to vascular spasm of migraine
     - (5) Tumors

(6) Nuclear types—pareses of a single or a few extraocular muscles supplied by the oculomotor nerve in one or both eyes. There may or may not be pupillary disturbances (mydriasis, sluggish pupillary reaction) and paresis of accommodation. In tumors within or near the midbrain (pinealomas) there is a combination of isolated muscle pareses with vertical gaze palsy, possibly a disturbance of convergence, and retraction nystagmus (Parinaud's syndrome, Sylvian aqueduct syndrome, pineal syndrome)

B. Intracranial
(1) Rupture of aneurysm at base of brain—third nerve paralysis, pain about the face (fifth nerve) and headache
(2) Polyneuritis due to toxins such as alcohol, lead, arsenic, dinitrophenol poisoning, carbon disulfide poisoning, and carbon monoxide, or to diabetes mellitus, herpes zoster, or mumps
(3) Poliomyelitis
(4) Syphilis and tuberculosis, meningitis, or encephalitis
(5) Multiple sclerosis
(6) Subdural hematoma
(7) Temporal arteritis
(8) Ophthalmic migraine
(9) Rabies
(10) Meningococcic meningitis
(11) Myasthenia gravis—worse p.m.
(12) Diphtheria
(13) Botulism
(14) Amebic dysentery
(15) Dengue fever
(16) Smallpox vaccination
(17) Hepatitis

C. Lesions affecting exit of third nerve from the cranial cavity
(1) Cavernous sinus syndrome—paralysis of third, fourth, and sixth nerves with proptosis
a. Cavernous sinus thrombosis

b. Pituitary adenoma—lateral extension
c. Aneurysm
d. Carotid-cavernous fistula
e. Extension of nasopharyngeal tumor
f. Extension from lateral sinus thrombosis

(2) Superior orbital fissure syndrome—same as for cavernous sinus syndrome except exophthalmos less likely to occur and optic nerve involvement and miotic pupil more likely
a. Sphenoid sinus suppuration
b. Skull fractures or hemorrhage
c. Tumors such as sphenoid ridge meningioma, nasopharyngeal tumor, and metastatic carcinomas, rhabdomyosarcoma, chordoma, sarcoma
d. Aneurysm
e. Occlusion of superior ophthalmic vein

(3) Orbital apex—involvement of third, fourth, sixth, first division of fifth, and optic nerves. Proptosis common

D. Other
(1) Lupus erythematosus
(2) Hodgkin's disease
(3) Sarcoid
(4) Dengue fever
(5) Associated with aspirin poisoning

3. Management (difficult to correct)—try to find CNS cause
A. Recession and resection—Recess LR 10 to 12 mm and resect MR 10 to 14 mm. This is most helpful if there is a partial return of MR function.
B. Transplantation of superior oblique tendon—Recess LR 10 to 12 mm, resect MR 10 to 14 mm and transplant SO tendon to insert at MR insertion. Free SO tendon nasal to SR, remove from trochlea, and resect it sufficiently so that it is taut when attached at point of MR insertion. This may help to splint eye in straight-ahead position.
C. If SO transplant fails, recess all tissues on the temporal aspect of the globe to the level of the lateral bony orbital rim and then anchor the eye in the primary position by a Callahan suture.

D. Lateral conjunctival recession may be of value in long-standing cases particularly if conjunctival dimpling is present on forced duction test.

E. With a lower division paralysis, i.e., inferior rectus, inferior oblique, and medial rectus muscle palsy (usually from trauma), transplant superior rectus to medial rectus muscle, lateral rectus to inferior rectus muscle and tenectomize superior oblique muscle.

F. Treat ptosis after other ocular muscle defects have been corrected.

Dyer, J. A.: Atlas of Extraocular Muscle Surgery. Philadelphia, W. B. Saunders, 1970, p. 156.

Frueh, B. R. and Sandall, G. S.: Superior Oblique Transplantation in Third Nerve Paralysis. Ann. Ophthal. 6:297-301, 1974.

Helveston, E. M.: Atlas of Strabismus Surgery, St. Louis, C. V. Mosby, 1973, pp. 156-159.

Hepler, R. S. and Cantu, R. C. Aneurysms and Third Nerve Palsies. Arch. Ophthal. 77:604-608, 1967.

Metz, H. S. and Yee, D.: Third Nerve Palsy: Superior Oblique Transposition Surgery. Ann. Ophthal. 5:215-218, 1973.

Roy, F. H.: Ocular Differential Diagnosis, 2nd ed. Philadelphia, Lea & Febiger, 1975, pp. 134-136.

Rucker, C. W.: The Causes of Paralysis of the Third, Fourth, and Sixth Cranial Nerves. Amer. J. Ophthal. 61:1293, 1966.

Walsh, F. B. and Hoyt, W. F.: Clinical Neuro-Ophthalmology. Baltimore, Williams & Wilkins, 1969.

INTERNUCLEAR OPHTHALMOPLEGIA

1. Clinical characteristics
   A. Paralysis of medial rectus muscles on attempted conjugate lateral gaze without other evidence of third nerve paralysis due to involvement of medial longitudinal fasciculus
   B. Jerk nystagmus of the abducting eye and vertical nystagmus, usually on upward gaze
2. Differential diagnosis
   A. Bilateral
      (1) Multiple sclerosis

(2) Inflammation, as upper respiratory infection
(3) Neoplasms–usually medulloblastomas or infiltrative gliomas
(4) Myasthenia gravis
(5) Occlusive vascular disease
(6) Syphilis
(7) Arnold-Chiari malformation
(8) Pontine hematoma
(9) Trauma

B. Unilateral
(1) Vascular lesion–infarct of small branch basilar artery
(2) Tumors of the brain stem
(3) Multiple sclerosis
(4) Myasthenia gravis

3. Treatment–identify cause

Cogan, D. G.: Internuclear Ophthalmoplegia, Typical and Atypical. Arch. Ophthal. 84:583-589, 1970.

Cogan, D. G., Kubik, C. S., and Smith, W. L.: Unilateral Internuclear Ophthalmoplegia. Arch. Ophthal. 44:783, 1950.

Glaser, J. S.: Myasthenic Pseudo-internuclear Ophthalmoplegia. Arch. Ophthal. 75:363, 1966.

Koos, W. T., Sunder-Plassmonn, M., and Salak, S.: Successful Removal of a Large Intrapontine Hematoma. J. Neurosurg. 31:690-694, 1969.

Rich, J. R., Gregorius, F. K., and Hepler, R. S.: Bilateral Internuclear Ophthalmoplegia After Trauma. Arch. Ophthal. 92:66-68, 1974.

Roy, F. H.: Ocular Differential Diagnosis, 2nd ed. Philadelphia, Lea & Febiger, 1975, p. 147.

Stroud, M. H., et al.: Abducting Nystagmus in the Medial Longitudinal Fasciculus (MLF) Syndrome–Internuclear Ophthalmoplegia (INO). Arch. Ophthal. 92:2-5, 1974.

PSEUDOHYPERTROPIA—ocular appearance of hypertropia with no manifest deviation of the visual axis

1. Facial asymmetry with one eye placed higher than the other
2. Unilateral ptosis
3. Unilateral coloboma
4. Orbital asymmetry

Shaterian, P. T. and Weissman, I. L.: An unusual case of pseudostrabismus. Amer. Orthopt. J. 23:68-70, 1973.

HYPER ALGORITHM—upward deviation of eye under cover with alternate cover test*

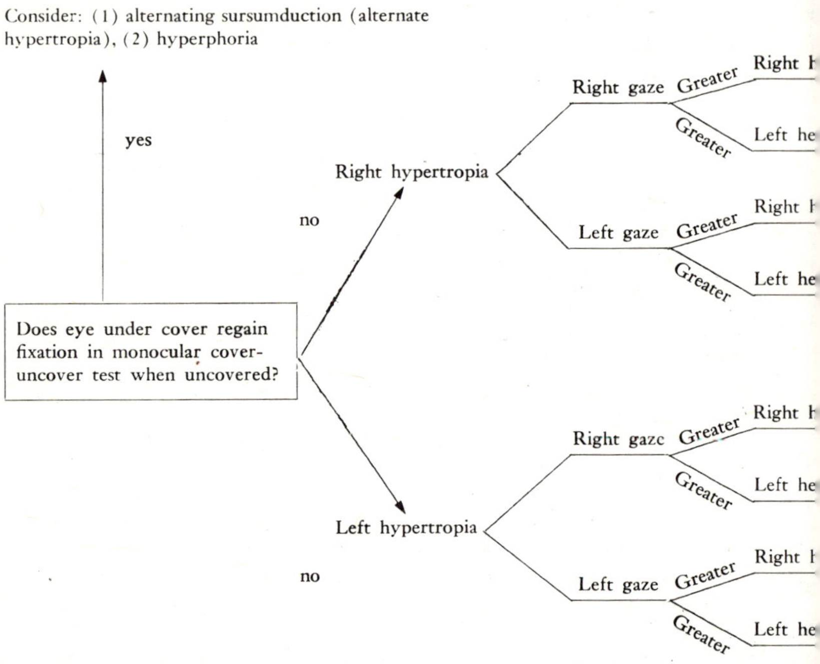

Consider: (1) alternating sursumduction (alternate hypertropia), (2) hyperphoria

yes

Does eye under cover regain fixation in monocular cover-uncover test when uncovered?

no

Right hypertropia

Right gaze Greater Right h
Greater Left he

Left gaze Greater Right h
Greater Left he

no

Left hypertropia

Right gaze Greater Right h
Greater Left he

Left gaze Greater Right h
Greater Left he

* Hardesty, H. H.: Diagnosis and Surgical Treatment of Paretic Vertical Muscles. Arch. Ophthal. 77:147-15
Parks, M. M.: Isolated Cyclovertical Muscle Palsy. Arch. Ophthal. 60:1027-1035, 1958.
Zipf, R. F. and Trokel, S. L.: Simulated Superior Oblique Tendon Sheath Syndrome Following Orbita Fracture. Amer. J. Ophthal. 75:700-705, 1973.

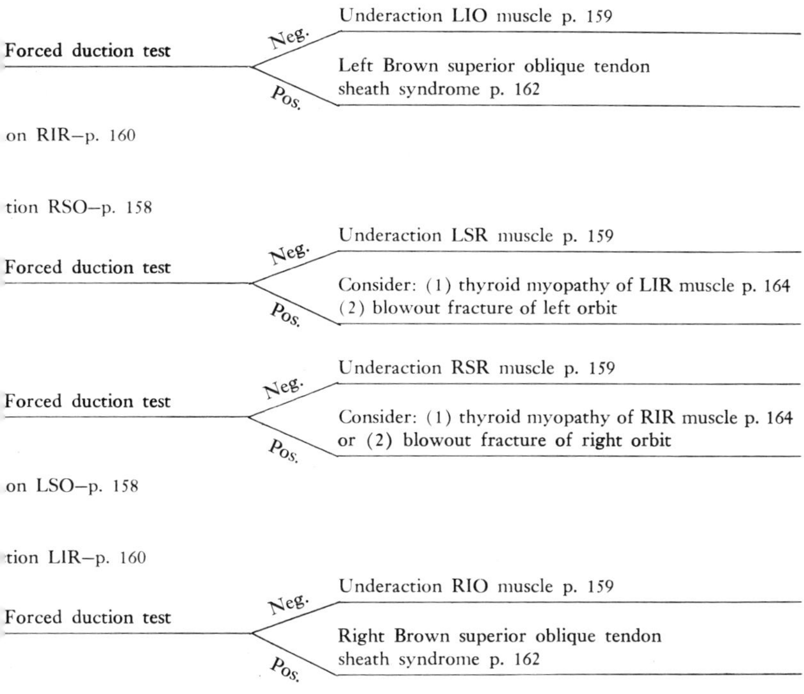

Forced duction test
- Neg. — Underaction LIO muscle p. 159
- Pos. — Left Brown superior oblique tendon sheath syndrome p. 162

on RIR—p. 160

tion RSO—p. 158

Forced duction test
- Neg. — Underaction LSR muscle p. 159
- Pos. — Consider: (1) thyroid myopathy of LIR muscle p. 164 (2) blowout fracture of left orbit

Forced duction test
- Neg. — Underaction RSR muscle p. 159
- Pos. — Consider: (1) thyroid myopathy of RIR muscle p. 164 or (2) blowout fracture of right orbit

on LSO—p. 158

tion LIR—p. 160

Forced duction test
- Neg. — Underaction RIO muscle p. 159
- Pos. — Right Brown superior oblique tendon sheath syndrome p. 162

HYPERTROPIA—one eye higher than the other

1. Apparent paralysis of elevation of one eye
   A. Dysthyroid ophthalmoplegia (noncongestive and congestive form)
   B. Myasthenia gravis
   C. Orbital floor fracture
   D. Abiotropic ophthalmoplegia (progressive nuclear ophthalmoplegia)
   E. Superior division, oculomotor nerve paresis
   F. Unilateral double elevator palsy, congenital absence of superior rectus and inferior oblique muscles
   G. Myositis
      (1) "Collagen diseases"
      (2) Infectious myositis
      (3) Trichinosis
   H. Systemic amyloidosis with ocular muscle infiltration
   I. Vertical retraction syndrome
   J. Superior oblique tendon sheath syndrome (Brown's) (see p. 162)

2. Apparent paralysis of elevation both eyes
   A. Physiological in older individuals
   B. Parinaud's syndrome–paralysis of vertical gaze due to lesion of superior colliculus, as pineal gland tumor
   C. Nuclear aplasia
   D. Progressive supranuclear palsy

3. Skew deviation due to lesion of central nervous system–one eye is above the other; may be the same for all directions of gaze or vary in different directions of gaze
   A. Unilateral labyrinthine disease
   B. Cerebellar tumors such as astrocytomas and medulloblastomas
   C. Acoustic neuromas
   D. Vascular accidents of pons and cerebellum such as thrombosis of cerebellar and pontine arteries
   E. Unilateral internuclear ophthalmoplegia (see internuclear ophthalmoplegia, p. 150) and less frequently bilateral internuclear ophthalmoplegia

   F. Compressive lesions such as platybasia and Arnold-Chiari malformation, brain stem arteriovenous malformations

4. Nonparalytic hypertropia
   A. Abnormal insertion of muscles
   B. Abnormal fascial attachments
   C. Complications of systemic diseases—myasthenia gravis, multiple sclerosis, thyrotoxicosis, orbital tumors, and brain stem disease

5. Paralytic hypertropia—isolated cyclovertical muscle palsy (see p. 156)

6. Double hyperphoria (alternating sursumduction)—fuses but cover test shows alternating hyperphoria

7. Apparent bilateral paralysis of down gaze
   A. Huntington's chorea
   B. Parkinsonism
   C. Early onset of progressive supranuclear palsy
   D. Head trauma
   E. Mumps, encephalitis
   F. Bilateral lesions medial and dorsal to red nuclei

Cogan, D. G.: Neurology of the Ocular Muscles, 2nd ed. Springfield, Charles C Thomas, 1969, pp. 134-135.

Jacobs, L., et al.: The Lesions Producing Paralysis of Downward but Not Upward Gaze. Arch. Neurol. 28:319-323, 1973.

Jampel, R. S. and Fells, P.: Monocular Elevation Paresis Caused by a Central Nervous System Lesion. Arch. Ophthal. 80:45, 1968.

Lessell, S., et al.: Brain Stem Arteriovenous Malformations. Arch. Ophthal. 86:255-259, 1971.

Pfaffenbach, D. D., Layton, D. D., and Kearns, T. P.: Ocular Manifestations in Progressive Supranuclear Palsy. Amer. J. Ophthal. 74: 1179-1189, 1972.

von Noorden, G. K. and Maumenee, A. E.: Atlas of Strabismus, 2nd ed. St. Louis, C. V. Mosby, 1973, pp. 154-160.

Walsh, F. B. and Hoyt, W. F.: Clinical Neuro-Ophthalmology. Baltimore, Williams & Wilkins, 1969.

ISOLATED CYCLOVERTICAL PALSY—superior and inferior rectus and superior and inferior oblique muscles moving the eye in a vertical plane. An abnormality of one of these muscles manifested as an isolated cyclovertical palsy

1. Management
   A. Congenital–The motor nerve, cyclovertical muscle or its attachment are not normal. Patient after six months usually shows obvious vertical strabismus or torticollis or both. Cyclovertical muscle surgery is indicated as soon as possible, even by the age of one year if surgeon is confident about his surgical findings. Early surgery offers the most rational means of preventing amblyopia, suppression and helping to maintain fusion. In addition, it helps to prevent permanent musculoskeletal changes of torticollis, facial asymmetry and scoliosis.
   B. Acquired–Try to pin down specific etiology of the fourth nerve (commonest) or third nerve which seldom gives an isolated cyclovertical palsy (p. 147). Treatment during the first six months usually consists of waiting to determine the degree of spontaneous recovery. Specific surgical correction of the acquired strabismus seldom should be delayed after six months from onset. Only one muscle at a time should be operated on and the degree of improvement studied over a three-month period, after which the decision as to further surgery should be made.

2. Differential diagnosis of fourth nerve palsy
   A. Intracerebral
      (1) Thrombosis of nutrient vessels, including median penetrating branch of basilar artery to fourth nucleus
      (2) Hemorrhage in the roof of the midbrain
      (3) Aneurysm including direct involvement by posterior cerebral and superior cerebellar arteries
      (4) Tumors
      (5) Neonatal hypoxia
      (6) Nuclear type–trochlear paresis combined with a homolateral oculomotor paresis, occasionally in association with vertical gaze palsies, convergence spasm

or convergence palsy, and pupillary disturbances as seen in tumors of the roof of the midbrain or pinealomas (pineal syndrome)

B. Intracranial
   (1) Aneurysms, as of the posterior communicating artery
   (2) Hematomas, traumatic
   (3) Tumors including cerebellopontine angle tumor
   (4) Meningitis, encephalitis, polyneuritis; diabetes mellitus, herpes zoster, multiple sclerosis, myasthenia gravis

C. Lesions affecting exit of fourth nerve from the cranial cavity
   (1) Cavernous sinus syndrome—paralysis of third, fourth, and sixth nerves with proptosis
      a. Cavernous sinus thrombosis
      b. Pituitary adenoma, lateral extension
      c. Aneurysm
      d. Carotid-cavernous fistula
      e. Extension of nasopharyngeal tumor
      f. Extension from lateral sinus thrombosis
   (2) Superior orbital fissure syndrome—same as for cavernous sinus syndrome except exophthalmos less likely to occur and optic nerve involvement and miotic pupil more likely
      a. Sphenoid sinus suppuration
      b. Skull fractures or hemorrhage
      c. Tumors such as sphenoid ridge meningioma, nasopharyngeal tumor, and metastatic carcinomas

C. Orbital apex syndrome

D. Orbital lesions
   (1) Fracture of superior orbital rim
   (2) Sinusitis
   (3) Operations upon the frontal sinus in which there is trochlear displacement
   (4) Trochlear disturbance as in Paget's disease or hypertrophic arthritis
   (5) Adherence syndrome—adhesions between the superior rectus and superior oblique muscles

(6) Abnormal insertion of superior oblique muscle or abnormal fascial attachments

(7) Idiopathic

3. Specific characteristics and surgical management—A weakening procedure is the operation of choice in 90% of the cases. With a compensatory head tilt, surgery should be directed to the paretic eye.

A. Underaction of the superior obliques—one of the most frequently involved vertical acting muscles. Look for the etiology of fourth nerve paresis or paralysis (see p. 156). With a right superior oblique palsy one would expect chin depression, a left head tilt, a left head turn and a right hypertropia which increases in left gaze and right head tilt. Vertical prisms of value in bilateral superior oblique paresis

Vertical prisms of value in bilateral superior oblique paresis

(1) Paresis of one superior oblique, for example RSO paresis

a. Right hypertropia greater in left up gaze than left down gaze—weaken RIO muscle by recession, disinsertion, or myotomy

b. Right hypertropia greater in left down gaze than left up gaze—tuck RSO (maximum 24 mm)

c. Right hypertropia same in up, down and lateral left gaze and 20 △ or less—weaken RIO muscle by recession, tenotomy or myotomy. If second procedure is needed, tuck RSO (maximum 24 mm)

d. Right hypertropia same in up, down and lateral left gaze and 25 △ or more—weaken RIO by myotomy or recession and tuck RSO at same procedure

e. Right hypertropia 25 △ or greater in up, down and lateral left gaze, straight down and down right gaze—weaken RIO by myotomy, tenotomy or recession *and* tuck RSO (maximum 24 mm)

f. Right hypertropia 25 △ or more in down left, straight down and down right gaze—tuck RSO (maximum 24 mm) and tenotomize LSO

(2) Paresis of both superior obliques (overaction both IOs)

a. Initial procedure–weaken both IOs by myotomy, disinsertion or recession
b. Second procedure if needed–recess both IRs (maximum 4 mm)

B. Underaction of the inferior obliques*–uncommon, may be abnormally in the muscle and surrounding fascia, or bones. Congenital type more likely to have head tilt and retained binocular vision. A right inferior oblique muscle might demonstrate chin elevation, right head tilt and left head turn and a left hypertropia which increases in left gaze and left head tilt. May be associated with the A syndrome. Usually some weakness of the superior rectus elevating capacity. Binocular vision in lower field of vision requires no surgical correction. If there is an underaction of the right inferior oblique
(1) Antagonist–recession or tenotomy RSO, if obvious overaction RSO, vertical tropia equal up and down gaze, and the forced duction test under anesthesia is positive
(2) Yolk–recession LSR, no obvious contracture of RIO (4 mm maximum)
(3) Palsied muscle–resection RSR (6 mm maximum) paretic eye fixates
(4) Yolk antagonist–resection LIR (6 mm maximum)

C. Underaction of the superior rectus muscle–unilateral or bilateral and frequently associated with congenital blepharoptosis. With a right superior rectus muscle palsy, the individual could have a right or left head tilt, right head turn and chin elevation and a left hypertropia which increases in right gaze and right head tilt. Most are congenital and patient may fixate with paretic eye. Evaluate ptosis and try to pin down specific etiology if possible (see p. 147). If there is an underaction of RSR
(1) Antagonist–recession RIR, vertical tropia equal up and down gaze, and forced duction test under anesthesia positive (4 mm maximum)

---

* The Brown superior oblique sheath syndrome must be ruled out in an underaction of the inferior oblique, by forced duction test. Brown's SO tendon sheath syndrome will have a positive forced duction test (p. 162). May have blowout fracture of orbit.

(2) Yolk–myotomy LIO, no obvious contracture RSR, paretic eye fixates and/or minimal limitation of elevation
(3) Palsied muscle–resection RSR (6 mm maximum) when nonparetic eye used for fixation
(4) Yolk antagonist–tucking LSO (10 mm maximum)

With marked paralysis of RSR, maximal recession RIR combined with resection of RSR and myotomy of the LIO would be needed.

D. Underaction of the inferior rectus muscle – isolated paresis uncommon and usually acquired from trauma. Right hypertropia which increases in right gaze and left head tilt and chin depression, right or left head tilt and a right head turn might occur with a right inferior rectus muscle palsy. May be unilateral or bilateral. With paretic RIR
(1) Antagonist–recession RSR, if obvious overaction RSR, vertical tropia equal up and down gaze, and the forced duction test under anesthesia positive (4 mm maximum)
(2) Yolk–tenotomy LSO, no obvious contracture RIR
(3) Palsied muscle–resection RIR (6 mm maximum)
(4) Yolk antagonist–tucking LIO (10 mm maximum)

With marked paralysis of RIR, maximal recession of RSR combined with resection of RIR may be necessary.

E. Double elevator palsy–superior rectus and inferior oblique of one eye involved. Unilateral, rare, and usually noted in orbital deformities, particularly Crouzon's disease. With right double elevator palsy
(1) Paretic (right) eye fixates – tuck RIO (10 mm maximum) and LIR resection (6 mm maximum)
(2) Nonparetic (left) eye fixates–tuck RIO (10 mm maximum) and recession RIR (4 mm maximum)

Burger, L. J., Kalvin, N. H., and Smith, J. L.: Acquired Lesions of the Fourth Cranial Nerve. Brain 93:567-574, 1970.

Dunlap, E. A.: Inferior Oblique Weakening: Recession, Myotomy, Myectomy or Disinsertion? Ann. Ophthal. 4:905-912, 1972.

Dyer, J. A.: Atlas of Extraocular Muscle Surgery. Philadelphia, W. B. Saunders, 1970, pp. 155-156.

Hardesty, H. H.: Diagnosis and Surgical Treatment of Paretic Vertical Muscles. Arch. Ophthal. 77:147-156, 1967.

Helveston, E. M.: A Two-Step Test for Diagnosing Paresis of a Single Vertically Acting Extraocular Muscle. Amer. J. Ophthal. 64:914-916, 1967.

Huber, A.: Eye Symptoms in Brain Tumors. St. Louis, C. V. Mosby, 1971, pp. 38-41.

Kass, M. A., Keltner, J. L., and Gay, A. J.: Total Third Nerve Paralysis. Arch. Ophthal. 87:107-109, 1972.

Khawom, E., Scott, A. B., and Jampolsky, A.: Acquired Superior Oblique Palsy. Arch. Ophthal. 77:761-768, 1967.

Knapp, P.: Diagnosis and Surgical Treatment of Hypertropia. 21:29-37, 1971.

Miller, M. T., Urist, M. J., Folk, E. R., and Chapman, L. I.: Superior Oblique Palsy Presenting in Late Childhood. Amer. J. Ophthal. 61: 1293, 1966.

Milstein, B. A. and Morretin, L. B.: Report of a Case of Sphenoid Fissure Syndrome Studied by Orbital Venography. Amer. J. Ophthal. 72:600-603, 1971.

Parks, M. M.: Isolated Cyclovertical Muscle Palsy. Arch. Ophthal. 60:1027, 1958.

Parks, M. M.: A Study of the Weakening Surgical Procedures for Eliminating Overaction of the Inferior Oblique. Trans. Amer. Ophthal. Soc. 69:163-187, 1971.

Roy, F. H.: Ocular Differential Diagnosis, 2nd ed. Philadelphia, Lea & Febiger, 1975, pp. 134-138.

Rucker, C. W.: The Causes of Paralysis of the Third, Fourth, and Sixth Cranial Nerves. Amer. J. Ophthal. 61:1293, 1966.

Sananman, M. L. and Weintroub, M. I.: Remitting Ophthalmoplegia Due to Rhabdomyosarcoma. Arch. Ophthal. 86:459-461, 1971.

Urist, M. J.: Unilateral Vertical Muscle Paresis with Secondary Vertical Deviations. Part II. Classification and Surgery. Amer. J. Ophthal. 57:1007-1037, 1964.

Urist, M. J.: A Technique For Recession of the Inferior Oblique Muscle. Arch. Ophthal. 87:198-201, 1972.

von Noorden, G. K. and Olson, C. L.: Diagnosis and Surgical Management of Vertically Incomitant Horizontal Strabismus. Amer. J. Ophthal. 60:434-442, 1965.

Walsh, F. B. and Hoyt, W. F.: Clinical Neuro-Ophthalmology. Baltimore, Williams & Wilkins, 1969.

Zipf, R. F. and Trokel, S. L.: Simulated Superior Oblique Tendon Sheath Syndrome Following Orbital Floor Fracture. Amer. J. Ophthal. 75:700-705, 1973.

BROWN'S SUPERIOR OBLIQUE TENDON SHEATH SYNDROME—congenital or acquired structural changes of the tendon or tendon sheath of the superior oblique muscle so that there is monocular limitation of elevation of the globe in adduction; demonstrated by restricted forced duction test

1. Types
   - A. Shortening of the tendon of the superior oblique muscle so that the thickened superior oblique muscle is closer to the trochlea and is unable to pass through the trochlea
   - B. Thickening of the tendon, resulting in impaired slippage through the trochlea
   - C. Congenital anomalous insertion of the superior oblique tendon
   - D. Acquired superior oblique tendon sheath syndrome–surgical tuck of the superior oblique muscle medially to the superior rectus muscle
   - E. An innervational abnormality in which the antagonist inferior oblique and superior oblique both are innervated. This can be demonstrated on electromyography (negative F.D. test)
   - F. Simulated Brown's syndrome
     - (1) Scar produced from superior nasal quadrant surgery
     - (2) Congenital or acquired restrictions affecting inferior orbital tissues, as blowout fracture
     - (3) Congenital anomalous check ligament from lateral orbit to insertion of inferior oblique
     - (4) Infection in the region of the trochlea or swelling of the superior oblique tendon restricting passage through the trochlea

2. Clinical characteristics–Usually there is fusion in the primary position and in the down position. The abnormality is worse on up gaze. The eye may demonstrate a nose dive in elevation if the eye is moved from abduction to adduction. May have lid elevation in field of IO resembling a paralysis. The chin may be elevated, or the head can be turned away from the field of action of the inferior oblique. For example, with a right superior oblique tendon sheath syndrome a left head turn (face turn) would be present and possibly a right head

tilt. Binocular vision is maintained, there is usually good equal vision, NRC, good range of fusion and stereopsis.

3. Diagnostic test—Forced duction test demonstrates in most types of the superior oblique tendon sheath syndrome a tight movement when the eye is moved up and medial and sometimes a clicking noise as the tight tendon is moved through the trochlea.

4. Treatment
   A. None if binocular single vision is present in the primary and down position and there is no cosmetic defect
   B. Surgery if there is a significant esotropia in the primary position or a major cosmetic defect, as head tilt or turn. Surgery consists of cutting superior oblique sheath and tucking inferior oblique tendon (maximum 10 mm) or sometimes in lengthening the tendon or tenotomizing the superior oblique. Knapp procedure—suture eye up and in with Supramyd and collagen suture, tie through lids and leave 5 to 10 days. Passive forced duction test during surgery delineates amount of restriction remaining.

Billet, E.: Superior Fascial Syndrome. J. Pediat. Ophthal. 4:47-51, 1967.

Brown, H. W.: Superior Oblique Tendon Sheath Syndrome. Strabismus-Ophthalmic Symposium. St. Louis, C. V. Mosby, 1950, p. 219.

Goldstein, J. H.: Intermittent Superior-Oblique-Tendon-Sheath Syndrome. Amer. J. Ophthal. 67:960-962, 1969.

Helveston, E. M.: Atlas of Strabismus Surgery. St. Louis, C. V. Mosby, 1973, pp. 110-111.

Sanford-Smith, J. H.: Intermittent Superior Oblique Tendon Sheath Syndrome: A Case Report. Brit. J. Ophthal. 53:412-417, 1969.

Zipf, R. F. and Trokel, S. L.: Simulated Superior Oblique Tendon Sheath Syndrome Following Orbital Floor Fracture. Amer. J. Ophthal. 75:700-705, 1973.

EXTERNAL OPHTHALMOPLEGIA (ocular muscle dystrophy)

1. Clinical characteristics—Slowly progressive ophthalmoplegia with multiple muscle involvement. No diplopia. Up gaze

usually most paretic. Pupils have normal direct and consensual light reflex. Age of onset is 30 to 60 years with autosomal dominant inheritance. May be associated with ophthalmoplegia of facial, neck muscles, retinal degeneration, and cerebellar ataxia.

2. Treatment—When no diplopia and cosmetically straight no treatment. Fresnel prisms may be used up to 20 △ deviation. Ptosis crutch may be helpful with ptosis. Surgery should be cautiously done.

Carlow, T. J. and Falls, H. F.: Idiopathic Progressive External Ophthalmoplegia. J. Pediat. Ophthal. 10:210-216, 1973.

Daroff, R. E.: Progressive External Ophthalmoplegia. Arch. Ophthal. 82:845-850, 1969.

Koerner, F. and Schlote, W.: Chronic Progressive External Ophthalmoplegia. Arch. Ophthal. 88:155-166, 1972.

Metz, H. S. and Cohen, M.: Progressive External Ophthalmoplegia. Ann. Ophthal. 5:775-778, 1973.

Walsh, F. B. and Hoyt, W. F.: Clinical Neuro-Ophthalmology, 3rd ed. Baltimore, Williams & Wilkins, 1969, pp. 1254-1257.

THYROID OCULAR MYOPATHY

1. Characteristics—Any of the extraocular muscles may become fibrotic and inelastic but this occurs most frequently with the inferior rectus and medial rectus. Adhesions between the ocular muscles and adjacent structures may severely impede elevation of the globe. Paralysis of the elevators is ruled out by a positive forced duction test.

2. Treatment—Wait until disease process has stabilized.
   A. If a IR is contracted recess it (maximum 4.5 mm); if a MR is contracted recess it (maximum 10 mm); if a SR is contracted, recess it (maximum 4.5 mm) and resect the IR and dissect the IR away from the IO as far posteriorly as possible to prevent retraction of the lid.
   B. Base operation on muscles obviously affected; if proper alignment is not obtained, wait 6 months before reopera-

tion. If results of the initial operation are obviously inadequate, one may reoperate on the same muscles within a few days. Usually it is best to increase the resection rather than the recession, since the latter was maximal at the first operation.

Caygill, W. M.: Excyclotropia in Dysthyroid Ophthalmopathy. Amer. J. Ophthal. 73:437-441, 1972.

Dyer, J. A.: Atlas of Extraocular Muscle Surgery. Philadelphia, W. B. Saunders, 1970, pp. 156-157.

Mein, J.: The Orthoptic Management of Exophthalmic Ophthalmoplegia. Amer. Orthopt. J. 18:52-65, 1968.

Pratt-Johnson, J. A., et al.: Surgical Treatment of Dysthyroid Restriction Syndromes. Canad. Ophthal. 7:405-412, 1972.

Schimek, R. A.: Surgical Management of Ocular Complications of Graves' Disease. Arch. Ophthal. 87:655-664, 1972.

von Noorden, G. K. and Maumenee, A. E.: Atlas of Strabismus, 2nd ed. St. Louis, C. V. Mosby, 1972, p. 166.

OCULAR MYASTHENIA GRAVIS

Extraocular muscles are involved in myasthenia gravis in a high percentage of cases. Ocular symptoms include ptosis, headache, asthenopia, and diplopia. One or more extraocular muscles may be weak. There may be presynaptic chemical abnormality which may be susceptible to immunological influence.

1. Classification (Osserman)
   - A. Neonatal—transient in infants of myasthenic mothers
   - B. Juvenile—may be familial, frequently stationary eye findings
   - C. Adult—myasthenia localized to the eyes. If there is no spread within a few years to other muscles, usually the disease does not progress. Frequently, increasingly severe systemic involvement, at least at onset
2. Diagnosis—high degree of suspicion by ophthalmologist
   - A. History—easy fatigability, acquired ptosis and acquired extraocular muscle palsy

B. Lid twitch sign (Cogan)—if after looking down the eyes are moved to the primary position, the upper lid twitches upward sometimes more than once. On horizontal gaze, there may be a brief flutter of the ptotic lid

C. Tensilon (10 mg/cc)
   (1) 0.2 cc (2 mg) I.V. in 15 to 30 seconds—needle left in place
   (2) No reaction after 45 seconds—give additional 0.8 cc (8 mg) I.V.
   (3) Cholinergic reaction as skeletal muscle fasciculations and increased muscle weakness—give 0.4 to 0.5 mg atropine I.V.
   (4) Positive reaction—decrease in ptosis or increase in muscle function seen in alignment, rotation, Lanchester red-green test, or Maddox rod test. Electromyography is a simple and nonpainful test which can be done even in children

3. Treatment—isolated extraocular muscle palsies frequently are resistant to treatment. The side effects of treatment may be so annoying that the patient prefers the disease. Many ophthalmologists prefer not to assume responsibility for treatment

   A. Neostigmine bromide (Prostigmin)—15 mg four times a day for mild myasthenia. If uncontrolled in several weeks combine with pyridostigmine (Mestinon) timespan one in the morning for two weeks and then one morning and night for two weeks. If not controlled on a combination of Prostigmin and Mestinon in about six weeks, usually the ocular myasthenia gravis will not be controlled by medical management
   B. Ambenonium chloride (Mytelase)
   C. Ephedrine sulfate—25 mg t.i.d.
   D. Demecarium bromide (Humorsol)—topical
   E. Prisms including conjugate-oblique prisms—prisms acting in the same direction, combined prisms acting disjunctively
      Example:
      O.D. 10 △ B.D and 8 △ BO
      O.S. 10 △ B.D and 8 △ BO

F. Fresnel prisms
G. Ptosis crutch

Diamond, S.: Prism Management of Vertical Incomitance; Case Reports: Conjugate Prism Correction for Ocular Myasthenia. Trans. Pacif. Coast Otoophthal. Soc. 46:135, 1965.

Leopold, I. H., et al.: Local Administration of Anticholinesterase Agents in Ocular Myasthenia Gravis. Arch. Ophthal. 63:544-547, 1960.

Osserman, K. E. and Genkins, G.: Critical Re-appraisal of the Use of Edrophonium (Tensilon) Chloride Tests in Myasthenia Gravis and Significance of Clinical Classification. Ann. N. Y. Acad. Sci. 135: 312-334, 1966.

Retzloff, J. A., et al.: Lancaster Red-Green Test in Evaluation of Edrophonium Effect in Myasthenia Gravis. Amer. J. Ophthal. 67: 13-21, 1969.

Smith, J. L.: Therapy for Ocular Myasthenia Gravis. Amer. Acad. Ophthal. Sept. 20, 1973.

Walsh, F. B. and Hoyt, W. F.: Clinical Neuro-Ophthalmology, 3rd ed. Baltimore, Williams & Wilkins, 1969, pp. 1277-1297.

ABNORMAL RETINAL CORRESPONDENCE—a binocular activity in which a cortical rearrangement is present in a strabismus patient to permit fusion of similar images projected on noncorresponding retinal areas. Unilateral suppression and peripheral fusion

1. Diagnosis
   A. Worth 4-dot test at 15 cm
      (1) ARC–fuses 2 red on one retina and 3 green lights on the other; as lights recede sees only 2 red or 3 green lights
      (2) NRC–sees 5 lights simultaneously
      (3) No retinal correspondence–sees either 2 lights or 3 lights
   B. Bagolini striated glasses at 135 degree and 45 degree axis (see p. 104)
      (1) ARC–one light, X formed gap where scotoma is
      (2) NRC–2 lights, line through each
      (3) No retinal correspondence–one light and one streak, either 135 degree or 45 degree

2. Treatment
   A. Prophylaxis as proper optical correction, alternate occlusion to prevent development of ARC, and early surgery
   B. Preoperative and postoperative orthoptics to increase fusional amplitudes combined with surgery to help to convert ARC to NRC
   C. Occasionally no treatment if ARC is well established and cosmetically satisfactory, patient has no symptoms, and some binocular function is present at the subjective angle. Stimulation of the suppressed foveal area of little value

Ing, M., et al.: Early Surgery for Congenital Esotropia. Amer. J. Ophthal. 61:1419-1427, 1966.

Parks, M. M.: Management of Eccentric Fixation and ARC in Esotropia. In: Symposium on Horizontal Ocular Deviations (Manley, D. R., Ed.). St. Louis, C. V. Mosby, 1971, pp. 81-87.

ECCENTRIC FIXATION—usually associated with strabismus and advanced amblyopia

1. Diagnosis–visuoscope and any other instrument which locates extrafoveal location of image of regard
2. Treatment
   A. Pleoptics–occlusion of eccentrically fixating eye, then occlusion of preferred eye
   B. Occlusion of the preferred eye
   C. Spectacles if significant refractive error
   D. Usually, eccentric fixation eliminated prior to surgery if surgery is required
   E. Prognosis
      (1) Below 4 years of age–good
      (2) 4 to 8 years of age–poor
      (3) Over 8 years of age–very poor
   F. With anisometropia, occlusion therapy and a contact lens might be considered

Clements, D. B.: Treatment of Eccentric Fixation by the Use of a Red Filter. Brit. J. Ophthal. 52:929-931, 1968.

Hilton, G. F.: The Diagnosis of Eccentric Fixation with the Indirect Ophthalmoscope. Arch. Ophthal. 81:650-652, 1969.

Keiner, E. C. J. F.: Pathogenesis of Eccentric Fixation. Amer. J. Ophthal. 63:20-22, 1967.

Malik, S. R. K., Gupta, A. K., and Choudhry, S.: The Red Filter Treatment of Eccentric Fixation. Amer. J. Ophthal. 67:586-590, 1969.

Nawratzki, I. and Oliver, M.: Eccentric Fixation Managed with Inverse Prism. Amer. J. Ophthal. 71:549-552, 1971.

Parks, M. M. and Friendly, D. S.: Treatment of Eccentric Fixation in Children under Four Years of Age. Amer. J. Ophthal. 61:395-399, 1966.

Parks, M. M.: Management of Eccentric Fixation and ARC in Esotropia. In: Symposium on Horizontal Ocular Deviations (Manley, D. R., Ed.). St. Louis, C. V. Mosby, 1971, pp. 81-87.

SYNDROMES ASSOCIATED WITH STRABISMUS*

1. Albright's hereditary osteodystrophy (pseudohypoparathyroidism)—strabismus, refractory end-organ to parathyroid hormone with hypocalcemia and hyperphosphatemia
2. Apert's syndrome (acrocephalosyndactylic syndrome)—strabismus, nystagmus, exophthalmos, slant fissure, field defect, keratitis, optic atrophy; syndactylia
3. Bloch-Sulzberger disease (incontinentia pigmenti)—strabismus, nystagmus, cataract, optic nerve involvement; bullous skin eruptions and pigmentations
4. Crouzon's disease (craniofacial dysostosis)—nystagmus, strabismus, exophthalmos, visual loss, anterior segment involvement; prognathism, maxillar atrophy, deformity of anterior fontanel
5. Cytomegalic inclusion disease, congenital—strabismus, failure to thrive, mental retardation, microcephaly, chorioretinitis, and seizures
6. Down's disease (mongolism, trisomy 21)—strabismus, epicanthal folds, oblique palpebral fissures, protruding tongue, open mouth, mental retardation, muscular hypotonia

* This section from Geeraets (pp. 234-235), with modifications.

7. Ehlers-Danlos disease (fibrodysplasia elastica generalisata)—hypotony of extraocular muscles, strabismus, ptosis, hyperelastic skin, thin sclera and cornea, keratoconus, subluxated lens, retinopathy; cutaneous hyperelasticity, atrophic skin, excessive articular laxity
8. Ellis-van Crefeld syndrome (chondroectodermal dysplasia)—internal strabismus, congenital cataract, iris coloboma; polydactylia, skeletal and genital anomalies, congenital heart defects (50%)
9. Erb-Goldflam disease (myasthenia gravis)—strabismus, ptosis, diplopia; myasthenia gravis, muscle weakness
10. Hallermann-Streiff syndrome (oculomandibulodyscephaly)—nystagmus, strabismus, cataract, microphthalmia; malformations of skeleton, teeth anomalies, mental retardation
11. Hemifacial microsomia (otomandibular dysostosis)—strabismus, microphthalmia, iris and choroidal colobomata; microtia, macrostomia, failure of development of mandibular ramus and condyle
12. Hurler's disease (mucopolysaccharidosis [MPS] type I)—strabismus, ptosis, corneal opacity, optic nerve and retinal involvement; retarded development, dorsolumbar kyphosis, head deformities
13. Hydrocephalus, congenital—strabismus, increased head size, protruding eyes with deficiency in upward gaze; poor motor development, neurologic abnormalities, and mental retardation
14. Laurence-Moon-Bardet-Biedl syndrome — nystagmus, strabismus, ophthalmoplegia, visual field defect, optic nerve and retinal involvement; obesity, hypogenitalism, polydactylia, mental deficiency
15. Marfan's syndrome (dystrophia mesodermalis congenita)—nystagmus, strabismus, anterior segment and lens involvement; arachnodactylia, congenital heart defect, relaxed ligaments
16. Millard-Gubler syndrome—paralysis of sixth nerve, diplopia, strabismus; hemiplegia of arm and leg
17. Naegeli's syndrome (melanophoric nevus syndrome)—nystag-

mus, strabismus, papillitis, pseudoglioma; keratosis, pigmentary skin changes

18. Nevoid basal cell carcinoma syndrome—strabismus, nevoid basal cell carcinomas, jaw cysts, cataracts, glaucoma, coloboma, chalazions

19. Parry-Romberg disease (progressive facial hemiatrophy)—strabismus, enophthalmos, Horner's syndrome, ptosis, miosis; facial hemiatrophy (loss of subcutaneous tissue)

20. Pierre Robin syndrome—strabismus; micrognathia, glossoptosis, cleft palate, respiratory distress

21. Prader Willi syndrome (hypotonia—obesity syndrome)— strabismus; obesity, hypogonadism, short stature, hypotonia, mental retardation, diabetes mellitus

22. Pseudohypoparathyroidism (Seabright-Bantam syndrome)—strabismus; obesity, short stature, tetany, mental retardation

23. Ring chromosome 18—strabismus, ptosis; mental retardation, microcephaly, low-set ears, deafness

24. Rubella, congenital—strabismus, microphthalmia, cataracts, glaucoma; congenital heart disease, deafness, mental/motor retardation

25. Rubinstein-Taybi syndrome—strabismus, antimongoloid slant of lid fissure, epicanthus, highly arched brows, refractive error; broad thumbs and toes, abnormal facial features, motor and mental retardation

26. Smith-Lemli-Opitz syndrome—strabismus, ptosis; mental retardation, skeletal and genital abnormalities, epicanthal folds

27. Supravalvular aortic stenosis syndrome (infantile hypercalcemia with mental retardation)—strabismus; infantile hypercalcemia, supravalvular aortic stenosis, mental retardation, "elfin-like" facies

28. Turner's syndrome (gonadal dysgenesis)—strabismus; short stature, webbing and/or shortening of neck, absence of secondary sexual characteristics, broad bridge of nose, epicanthal folds, low-set ears

29. GML-Gangliosidosis—esotropia, nystagmus, optic atrophy; large head, coarse features, hypotonia, peripheral edema
30. Francois dyscephalic syndrome—dyscephaly with bird's head, microphthalmia, congenital cataracts, nystagmus; dental anomalies, proportioned dwarfism
31. Seckel's bird-headed dwarfism—microcephaly, narrow beaked nose, narrow face, mental retardation
32. DeLange syndrome—synophrys and telecanthus, blue sclera, strabismus, nystagmus, myopia, ptosis
33. Leigh's disease (subacute necrotizing encephalomyelopathy)
34. Short-arm deletion chromosome 18 – web neck, ptosis, cataracts, hypertelorism, strabismus
35. Noonan's syndrome (male Turner's syndrome): antimongoloid slant, hypertelorism, epicanthal folds, exophthalmos, high myopia, keratoconus, posterior embryotoxon
36. Chromosome 18 partial short-arm deletion syndrome (Wolf's syndrome)—iris and/or retinal coloboma, hypertelorism, epicanthus, strabismus, microcephaly, hydrocephalus, seizures
37. Nevus sebaceus of Jadassohn—antimongoloid lid, dermoid limbus, coloboma iris-choroid, nystagmus, external oculomotor palsy (unilateral), thickening of bones of orbit, coloboma lids
38. Craniocarpotarsal dysplasia (Freeman-Sheldon syndrome, whistling face syndrome)—antimongoloid lid fissures, esotropia, mild ptosis, high skull, protruding lips as in whistling, receding chin, and high palate
39. Cri du chat syndrome (cat cry)—short-arm deletion of chromosome 5, strabismus, decreased tearing, hypertelorism, tortuosity of retinal vessels
40. Congenital hypothyroidism
41. Cockayne's syndrome

Emery, J. M., et al.: GML-Gangliosidosis: Ocular and Pathological Manifestations. Arch. Ophthal. 85:177-187, 1971.

Francois, J. and Pierard, J.: The Francois Dyscephalic Syndrome and Skin Manifestations. Amer. J. Ophthal. 71:1241-1250, 1971.

Geeraets, W. J.: Ocular Syndromes. Philadelphia, Lea & Febiger, 1969, pp. 234-235.

Gellis, S. S. and Feingold, M.: Atlas of Mental Retardation. Washington, U. S. Printing Office, 1968.

Goodman, R. M. and Gorlin, R. J.: The Face in Genetic Disorders. St. Louis, C. V. Mosby, 1970, pp. 38, 46, 146.

Haslam, R. H. and Wirtschafter, J. D.: Unilateral External Oculomotor Nerve Palsy and Nevus Sebaceous of Jadassohn. Arch. Ophthal. 87:293-300, 1972.

Howard, R. O. and Albert, D. H.: Ocular Manifestations of Subacute Necrotizing Encephalomyelopathy (Leigh's Disease). Arch. Ophthal. 86:386-393, 1972.

Howard, R. O.: Ocular Abnormalities in the Cri du Chat Syndrome. Amer. J. Ophthal. 73:949-954, 1973.

Johnson, R. V. and Kennedy, W. R.: Progressive Facial Hemiatrophy (Parry-Romberg Syndrome). Amer. J. Ophthal. 67:561, 1969.

Kirkland, R. T., et al.: Strabismus and Congenital Hypothryoidism. J. Pediat. 80:648-650, 1972.

Levenson, J. E., Crandall, B. F., and Sparkes, R. S.: Partial Deletion Syndromes of Chromosome 18. Ann. Ophthal. 3:756-760, 1971.

Milot, J. and Denoy, F.: Ocular Anomalies in DeLange Syndrome. Arch. Ophthal. 74:394-399, 1972.

Pearce, W. G.: Ocular and Genetic Features of Cockayne's Syndrome. Canad. J. Ophthal. 7:435-444, 1972.

Roy, F. H.: Dungan, T., and Fulow, C.: Infantile Hypercalcemia and Supravalvular Stenosis. J. Pediat. Ophthal. 8:188-194, 1971.

Roy, F. H.: Ocular Differential Diagnosis, 2nd ed. Philadelphia, Lea & Febiger, 1975, pp. 112-115.

Schwartz, D. E.: Noonan's Syndrome Associated with Ocular Abnormalities. Amer. J. Ophthal. 73:955-960, 1972.

Visual Field Problems

Visual Field Problems

CONTENTS

Visual Field Problems

INTRODUCTION

Most texts look at the diagnosis rather than the patient's problems. The two are usually not the same.

This material on visual fields was developed because many visual fields implicate nonocular problems. These are usually referred to a neurologist or neurosurgeon. Frequently the ophthalmologist gets that "bad-looking field" patient out of the office and does not lend his professional skill to the decision making. The algorithms on pages 189, 191, 193, 196, 197, 198, 199 have about an 80% accuracy in deciding the underlying problems. In addition, there are differential diagnosis lists on pages 182, 183, 184, 185, 187, 188, 189, 192, 194 to consider possibilities compatible with the patient's history and ocular examination. Ophthalmologists should consider themselves part of the team working out the patient's problems, and this material was designed to work toward this goal.

Great strides are being made in standardization of visual field examinations. Computerization of visual field examination has almost brought this examination into the realm of the routine ocular examination.

Assistance and suggestions were provided in the preparation of this material by Drs. Dennis Lucy, Sam Boellner, George Lucas, and Fritz Fraunfelder. Preparation of the manuscript and proof reading were ably provided by Mrs. Diane Butler, Mr. Steve Elrod, Mrs. Pat Baxter, and Mrs. Renee Massey.

PRESENTING VISUAL FIELD PROBLEMS (indications for visual fields)

1. Subjective
   A. "Unable to see to the side" or "holes in vision"
   B. Reading difficulties
      (1) Sees one letter better if looks at second one—may indicate scotoma
      (2) Reads test line backward—may indicate chiasmal lesion or bitemporal hemianopia
      (3) Leaves out part of letter, as C for O or F for E—may indicate tiny scotoma
   C. Difficulty with color vision
   D. Poor visual acuity (unexplained)
   E. Poor night vision
   F. Clumsiness, spills food at table or bumps into objects—may indicate homonymous hemianopia or inferior field defect
2. Objective
   A. Disc abnormalities of optic atrophy, papilledema, papillitis, retrobulbar neuritis and drusen
   B. Glaucoma—initial and follow-up
   C. Retinal abnormality, as retinal detachment or tumors
   D. Sudden-onset paralysis of extraocular muscles (third, fourth or sixth)

VISUAL FIELDS TESTING MODALITIES

1. Confrontation—best used for gross screening and pediatric, obtunded or dysphasic patients. Simple, inexpensive
   A. Target is presented serially in various quadrants of visual field
   B. Targets may be present in right and left fields simultaneously
   C. Small toys or pictures, small flashing lights or even the examiner's face may be used with the very young

2. Goldmann perimeter
   A. Tests both central and peripheral fields
   B. Reproducible results with cooperative patient with controlled background illumination and target intensity
   C. High cost (about $3,000)
   D. Difficult for technician to achieve consistent good results
3. Target screen
   A. Tests central 25 to 30 degrees
   B. Magnifies central defect by being farther away from screen
   C. Patient must wear full correction for the refractive error
   D. Wands may be B&L, Berens, or Lumiwand
4. Aimark perimeter—projection perimeter with targets of 1 to 10 mm, series of color filters, and neutral density gray filters
   A. Self-recording unit
   B. Patient may use finger for fixation with dense scotoma
   C. Good for testing peripheral defects

SPECIFIC FIELD DEFECTS

Pseudo-field Defect

1. Facial contour
   A. Prominent nose
   B. Bushy projecting eyebrows
   C. High cheekbones
   D. Ptosis or blepharochalasis
2. Corneal opacities
3. Lenticular opacities, especially if miotics are used. Depress fields and exaggerate existing scotoma
4. Aphakia without lens or with convex lens; little distortion with contact lens or intraocular acrylic lens
5. Dull patient—may be mentally defective, have toxemia, arteriosclerosis, cerebral tumor, brain abscess, or increased intracranial pressure

6. Pupillary size
   A. Miotic–decrease field especially with opacities of ocular media
   B. Drooping of upper lid over pupillary aperture–decrease field
7. Uncorrected refractive errors–correct presbyopia for distance testing
8. Head tilting–when the head is tilted toward left shoulder the right blind spot is elevated; when the head is tilted to the right shoulder the right blind spot is lowered
9. Environmental artifacts
   A. Reduction of illumination of screen and test objects
   B. Test object size if varied
   C. Standard distance of patient from screen
   D. Attention of patient
   E. Technique of examiner
10. Psychological artifacts
    A. Misunderstanding of test by patient
    B. Tiring of patient by prolonged testing
    C. Malingering–isopters at different distances are inconsistent
    D. Hysteria–spiral field defects may be found
11. Frame of glasses and segments of multifocal lenses

Reed, H.: The Essentials of Perimetry. New York, Oxford University Press, 1960, pp. 37, 66-69.

Bilateral Central Scotomas—bilateral macular defects with decreased visual acuity; the scotomas may be central or centrocecal

1. Bilateral macular lesions such as cysts or due to hemorrhage, edema, degeneration, detachment, hole, or infection
2. Bilateral optic nerve lesions
   A. Papillitis
   B. Retrobulbar neuritis
   C. Papilledema with macular edema
3. Toxic agents
   A. Tobacco

B. Ethyl alcohol
C. Methyl alcohol
D. Carbon disulfide
E. Halogenated hydrocarbons–methyl chloride, methyl bromide, iodoform, trichloroethylene
F. Aromatic amino- and nitro- compounds–aniline, nitrobenzene, trinitrotoluene
G. Drugs
   (1) Sedatives–barbiturates, ethchlorvynol, pheniprazine, disulfiram, opium, morphine
   (2) Anti-infective drugs–sulfanilamide, isoniazid, chloramphenicol
   (3) Miscellaneous drugs–digoxin, stramonium, thyroxin, ricin, apiol, nicotinic acid
H. Metals–lead, thallium, (inorganic) arsenic

4. Familial optic atrophy
5. Migraine–forerunner of visual auras
6. Occipital cortex lesions
7. Nutritional deficiency, as thiamine or vitamin B_{12} deficiency
8. Pernicious anemia
9. Diabetes mellitus

Cocke, J. G.: Chloramphenicol Optic Neuritis. Amer. J. Dis. Child, 114:424-426, 1967.

Duke-Elder, S. and Scott, G. I.: System of Ophthalmology, Vol. XII. St. Louis, C. V. Mosby, 1971, pp. 145-166.

Friedman, B.: Migraine: with Special Reference to Scintillating Scotoma. Eye Ear Nose Throat Monthly 50:52-58, 1971.

Harrington, D. O.: The Visual Fields, 3rd ed. St. Louis, C. V. Mosby, 1971.

Roy, F. H.: Ocular Differential Diagnosis, 2nd ed. Philadelphia, Lea & Febiger, 1975, pp. 499-500.

Enlargement of the Blind Spot

1. Papilledema
2. Papillitis
3. Glaucoma

4. Progressive myopia with a temporal crescent
5. Medullated nerve fibers
6. Drusen of the optic nerve
7. Coloboma of the optic nerve
8. Senility–senile halo
9. Early manifestation of other defect such as centrocecal scotoma or arcuate defect
10. Inferior conus
11. Juxtapapillary choroiditis
12. Inverted disc or nasally directed scleral canal

Drance, S. M.: The Visual Field in Glaucoma: Current Status. Trans. Amer. Acad. Ophthal. Otolaryng. 78:301-303, 1974.

Reed, H.: The Essentials of Perimetry. New York, Oxford University Press, 1960, pp. 69-70.

Roy, F. H.: Ocular Differential Diagnosis, 2nd ed. Philadelphia, Lea & Febiger, 1975, pp. 500-501.

Zuckerman, J.: Perimetry. Philadelphia, J. B. Lippincott, 1954.

Arcuate (Cuneate) Scotoma (Nerve Fiber Defect)—the scotoma follows the lines of the nerve fibers in the retina with the narrow end at the blind spot and broad end at horizontal raphe

1. Glaucoma
2. Vascular accident affecting the optic nerve
3. Acute bleeding episode
4. Drusen of optic nerve
5. Chorioretinitis juxtapapillaris
6. High myopia
7. Coloboma of the disc
8. Inferior conus
9. Supratraction
10. Ischemic optic neuropathy with splinter hemorrhage on optic disc
11. Chromophobe adenoma

Drance, S. M. and Begg, I. S.: Sector Hemorrhage: A Probable Acute Ischemic Disc Change. Canad. J. Ophthal. 5:137-141, 1970.

Drance, S. M.: The Glaucomatous Visual Field. Invest. Ophthal. 11: 85-97, 1972.

Harrington, D. O.: The Visual Fields, 3rd ed. St. Louis, C. V. Mosby, 1971.

Heilmann, K.: On the Reversibility of Visual Field Defects in Glaucoma. Trans. Amer. Acad. Ophthal. Otolaryng. 78:304-308, 1974.

Reed, H.: The Essentials of Perimetry. New York, Oxford University Press, 1960, p. 85.

Roy, F. H.: Ocular Differential Diagnosis, 2nd ed. Philadelphia, Lea & Febiger, 1975, pp. 501-502.

Trobe, J. D.: Chromophobe Adenoma Presenting with a Hemianopic Temporal Arcuate Scotoma. Amer. J. Ophthal. 77:388-392, 1974.

Unilateral Sector-shaped Defects—narrow end of scotoma characteristically touches the physiological blind spot

1. Optic disc involvement
   A. Secondary optic atrophy after choked disc (more on nasal side)
   B. Papillitis
   C. Glaucoma (early stages primarily nasal side)
2. Retina
   A. Juxtapapillary chorioretinitis
   B. Branch embolism of the central retinal artery
3. Optic nerve–between disc and chiasm
   A. Tumor
   B. Aneurysm
   C. Drusen

Huber, A.: Eye Symptoms in Brain Tumors, 2nd ed. St. Louis, C. V. Mosby, 1971, p. 83.

Knight, C. L. and Hoyt, W. F.: Monocular Blindness from Drusen of the Optic Disc. Amer. J. Ophthal. 73:890-892, 1972.

Peripheral Field Contraction—central vision present; patient may complain of poor night vision

1. Optic atrophy
2. Retinitis pigmentosa
3. Papillitis
4. Glaucoma
5. Hysteria

6. Retinitis–periphery of fundus
7. Choroiditis–periphery of fundus
8. Poisons
   A. Quinine
   B. Chloroquine
   C. Arsenic
   D. Salicylates
   E. Optochin
   F. Filix mas
   G. Carbon monoxide
   H. Thioridazine
   I. Oxygen
   J. Carbon tetrachloride
   K. Methyl iodide
   L. Acridine derivatives
   M. Ergot
   N. Aspidium and other vegetable derivatives
9. Many conditions in which night blindness occurs
10. Drusen of optic disc
11. Double homonymous hemianopsia–If the macular sparing in one homonymous hemianopsia is larger than that in the other, the spared central portion of the field will have small vertical steps, above and below fixation where the two areas of macular sparing do not quite coincide
    A. Stroke or infarction of occipital lobe
    B. Cortical blindness with damage to occipital lobe and macular recovery
       (1) Trauma
       (2) Anoxia
       (3) Carbon monoxide poisoning
       (4) Cerebral angiography
       (5) Cardiac arrest
       (6) Exsanguination
12. Frontal lobe tumors
13. General apathy in a lackadaisical subject
14. Chronic atrophic papilledema

15. Unilateral concentric construction excluding diseased retina or glaucoma–suggests lesion of optic nerve and chiasm
    A. Tumor optic nerve
    B. Meningioma tuberculum sellae, sphenoid ridge or the olfactory groove

Duke-Elder, S. and Scott, G. I.: System of Ophthalmology, Vol. XII. St. Louis, C. V. Mosby, 1971, pp. 145-166.

Harrington, D. O.: The Visual Fields, 3rd ed. St. Louis, C. V. Mosby, 1971, pp. 125-126, 220-224.

Huber, A.: Eye Symptoms in Brain Tumors, 2nd ed. St. Louis, C. V. Mosby, 1971, pp. 81-82.

Knight, C. L. and Hoyt, W. F.: Monocular Blindness from Drusen of the Optic Disc. Amer. J. Ophthal. 73:890-892, 1972.

Roy, F. H.: Ocular Differential Diagnosis, 2nd ed. Philadelphia, Lea & Febiger, 1975, pp. 503-504.

Altitudinal Hemianopia—defective vision or blindness in the upper or lower horizontal half of the visual field, may be unilateral or bilateral; the unilateral field defect is prechiasmal

1. Superior or inferior retinal artery obstruction–unilateral
2. Glaucomatous cupping–usually greatest in lower portion of optic nerve, giving superior altitudinal hemianopia; associated especially with low-tension glaucoma
3. Optic nerve lesions as papilledema and atrophy of tabes
4. Injury to the optic nerve due to torsion, edema, or shearing of the small vessels supplying the optic nerve
5. Coloboma of optic nerve
6. Sclerotic plaques of internal carotid artery or anterior cerebral arteries–pressure of plaques on optic nerve resulting in inferior altitudinal hemianopia
7. Fusiform aneurysms (arteriosclerotic or congenital)–may produce inferior altitudinal hemianopia by pressure against the lateral halves of the optic chiasm or nerve
8. Lesion pressing the chiasm upward against the superior margin of the optic foramen

9. Olfactory groove meningioma extending posteroinferior to compress the intracranial portion of the optic nerve
10. Trauma to or vascular insufficiency of occipital lobe–inferior altitudinal hemianopia when the upper lips of both calcarine fissures are damaged; superior altitudinal hemianopia when the lower lips of both calcarine fissures are damaged
11. Anemia–produces bilateral inferior altitudinal hemianopia
12. Exsanguination
13. Ischemic optic neuropathy

Cogan, D. G.: Neurology of the Visual System, 3rd ed. Springfield, Charles C Thomas, 1966, pp. 31, 137, 185, 188, 224.

Drance, S. M., et al.: Studies of Factors Involved in the Production of Low Tension Glaucoma. Arch. Ophthal. 89:457-465, 1973.

Harrington, D. O.: The Visual Fields, 3rd ed. St. Louis, C. V. Mosby, 1971.

Roy, F. H.: Ocular Differential Diagnosis, 2nd ed. Philadelphia, Lea & Febiger, 1975, pp. 505-506.

Binasal Hemianopia—defects in nasal half of visual fields, usually incomplete, due to lateral involvement of the chiasm; presupposes bilateral lesions

1. Chiasmic arachnoiditis, postneuritic optic atrophy, and bilateral retrobulbar neuritis of multiple sclerosis
2. Drusen of optic nerve
3. Fusiform aneurysms–arteriosclerotic or congenital–of internal carotid artery
4. Sclerotic plaques of internal carotid artery or anterior cerebral arteries
5. Pituitary tumor with third ventricle dilation pushing laterally
6. Symmetrical lesions in the temporal halves of both retinas as severe retinal edema associated with diabetic retinopathy
7. Nasal quadrant peripheral depression of glaucoma–bilateral and reasonably symmetrical
8. Bilateral occipital lesion (thrombosis)

9. Trauma
10. Severe exsanguination

Cogan, D. G.: Neurology of the Visual System, 3rd ed. Springfield, Charles C Thomas, 1966, pp. 150, 188, 210, 217, 224.

Duke-Elder, S. and Scott, G. I.: System of Ophthalmology, Vol. XII. St. Louis, C. V. Mosby, 1971, pp. 292-293.

Harrington, D. O.: The Visual Fields, 3rd ed. St. Louis, C. V. Mosby, 1971, pp. 123-124.

Roy, F. H.: Ocular Differential Diagnosis, 2nd ed. Philadelphia, Lea & Febiger, 1975, pp. 506-507.

Bitemporal Hemianopic Field Defect (bilateral temporal visual field defect)—usually incomplete due to pressure in optic chiasm; if complete almost invariably demonstrates subnormal visual acuity (80% accurate)

1. Most common

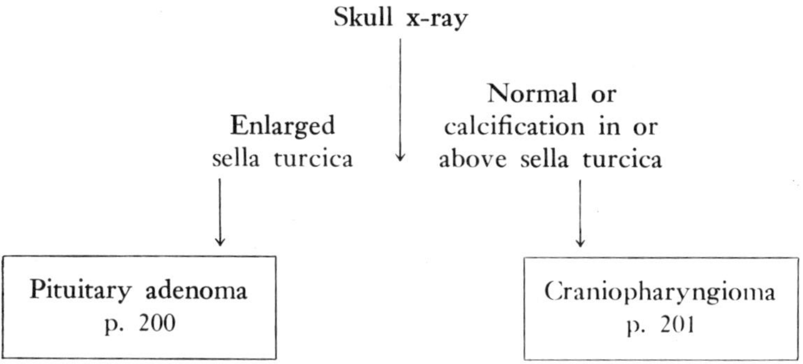

2. Differential diagnosis
   A. Chiasmal lesions
      (1) Vascular lesions
         a. Arteriosclerosis
         b. Arterial compression
         c. Thrombosis of the carotid artery
         d. Intracranial aneurysms as congenital, endocardial emboli, traumatic, atheromatic, or syphilitic (especially intrasellar) aneurysms

(2) Inflammatory lesions
- a. Chiasmal neuritis
- b. Basal meningitis including chronic chiasmal arachnoiditis, syphilitic, tuberculous, actinomycotic and cysticercal

(3) Tumors of the chiasma
- a. Primary tumors including gliomas in childhood
- b. Secondary tumors (rare) including meningioma, retinoblastoma, pinealoma, and ependymoma

B. Pituitary lesions

(1) Pituitary hyperplasia

(2) Pituitary tumors (see p. 200)
- a. Adenoma
  - 1) Chromophobe adenoma–varies from no endocrine symptoms to panhypopituitarism (most common type of pituitary tumor)
  - 2) Acidophilic adenoma–varies from gigantism to acromegaly
  - 3) Basophilic adenoma – hyperadrenalism (Cushing's disease) (rare)
- b. Adenocarcinoma (rare)
- c. Metastatic tumors (rare) as from breast

C. Perisellar lesions

(1) Suprasellar tumors
- a. Craniopharyngioma – manifestations may include diabetes insipidus, infantilism, and calcification of hypophyseal-pituitary region (see p. 201)
- b. Suprasellar meningioma
- c. Cholesteatoma
- e. Epidermoid
- f. Teratoma
- g. Pinealoma
- h. Lymphoblastoma
- i. Tumors of the frontal lobe including porencephaly (cystic cavity in brain substance) and glioma
- j. Tumors of the third ventricle and internal hydrocephalus as glioma and ependymoma

(2) Presellar tumors
 a. Meningioma of the olfactory groove
 b. Neuroblastoma of the olfactory groove
(3) Parasellar tumors
 a. Meningioma of the sphenoid ridge
 b. Tumors of the sphenoid bone including osteochondroma, sarcoma, anaplastic carcinoma
 c. Tumors of the basal meninges
 d. Injuries to the chiasmal pathway as traumatic
 e. Migraine
 f. Sudden onset without apparent cause
  1) Disseminated sclerosis
  2) Arteriosclerotic or giant cell arteritic occlusion of nutrient vessels of the chiasm in elderly patients

Cogan, D. G.: Neurology of the Visual System, 3rd ed. Springfield, Charles C Thomas, 1966, pp. 217, 222, 224, 228, 233, 239.

Duke-Elder, S. and Scott, G. I.: System of Ophthalmology, Vol. XII. St. Louis, C. V. Mosby, 1971, pp. 299-395.

Roy, F. H.: Ocular Differential Diagnosis, 2nd ed. Philadelphia, Lea & Febiger, 1975, pp. 507-508.

Walsh, F. B. and Hoyt, W. F.: Clinical Neuro-Ophthalmology, 3rd ed. Baltimore, Williams & Wilkins, 1969, pp. 69-75, 730, 1974.

Blindness in One Eye and Temporal Visual Field Defect in Other Eye (80% accurate)

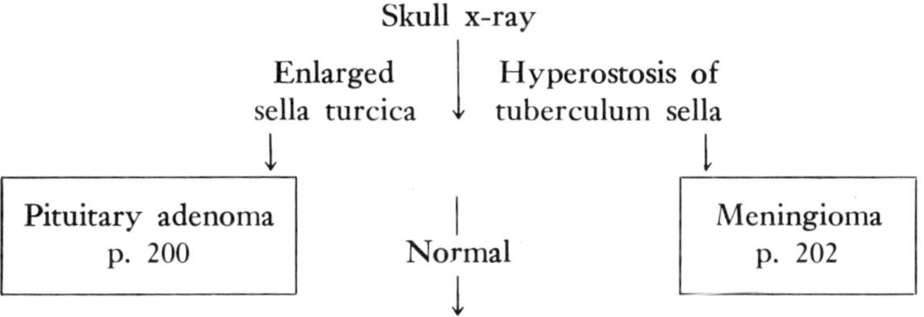

Youth—craniopharyngioma p. 201
Adult—pituitary adenoma p. 200
or
meningioma p. 202

Homonymous Quadrantanopsia — one quadrant involved; upper or lower and right or left visual fields

1. Superior homonymous quadrantanopsia
   A. Temporal lobe–incongruous (p. 197)
   B. Inferior lip of the calcarine fissure–congruous (p. 199)
2. Inferior homonymous quadrantanopsia
   A. Superior radiation in parietal lobe–incongruous (p. 198)
   B. Upper lip of the calcarine fissure in the occipital lobe–congruous (p. 199)

Harrington, D. O.: The Visual Fields, 3rd ed. St. Louis, C. V. Mosby, 1971, p. 121-123.

Crossed Quadrantanopsia—upper quadrant of one visual field is lost along with the lower quadrant of the opposite visual field

1. Chiasm compression from lesion below compressing it against contiguous arterial structure
2. Glaucoma
3. Inflammatory lesion as choroiditis juxtapapillaris
4. Asymmetrical homonymous hemianopsia such as vascular lesion of the upper lip of the calcarine area on one side and the lower lip of the opposite calcarine cortex

Harrington, D. O.: The Visual Fields, 3rd ed. St. Louis, C. V. Mosby, 1971, p. 124.

Homonymous Hemianopia—visual field defect on the same side in each eye, i.e., with temporal defect left eye and nasal defect right eye, the lesion is on the right side, posterior to the optic chiasm (80% accurate)

1. Most common

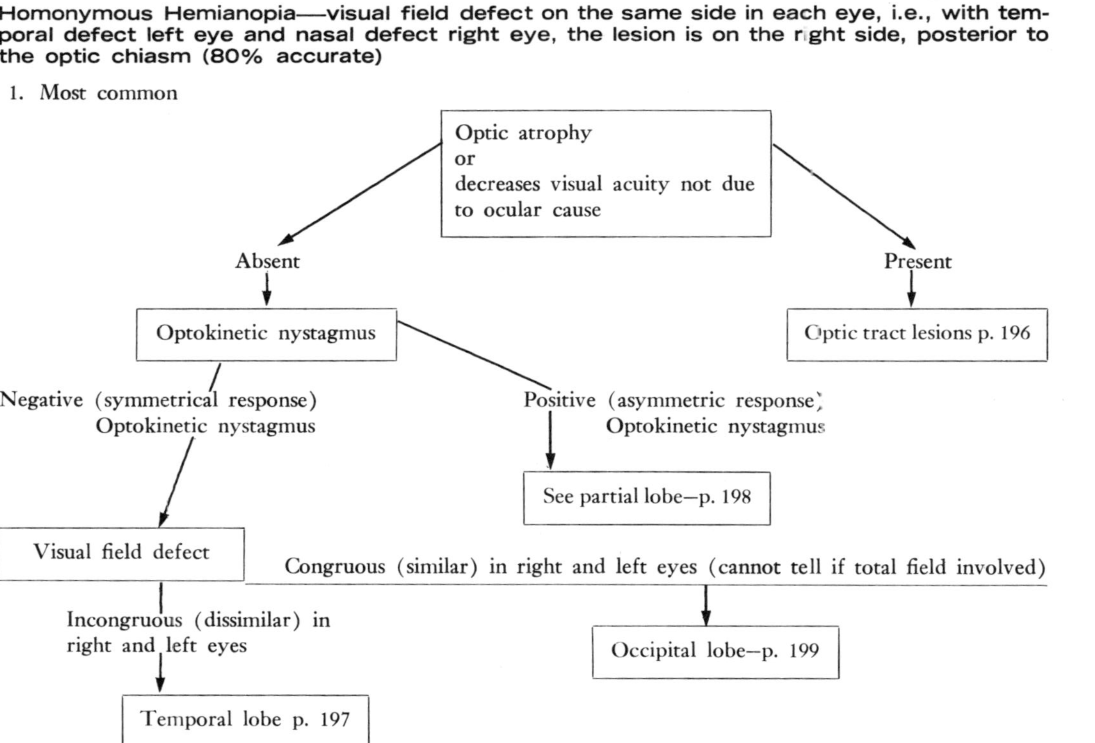

2. Differential diagnosis
   A. Optic tract lesions
      (1) Saccular aneurysms of internal carotid or posterior communicating artery (see p. 202)
      (2) Pituitary adenomas and craniopharyngiomas (most common); nasopharyngeal carcinomas, chordomas, infundibulomas, and gliomas (less common)
      (3) Demyelinative disease–retrobulbar, multiple sclerosis, and Schilder's disease
      (4) Trauma
      (5) Migraine
   B. Temporoparietal lesions–those of temporal lobe manifest initially in the upper visual fields, those of parietal lobe manifest first in the lower visual fields
      (1) Vascular lesions–sudden onset
         a. Thrombosis–premonitory symptoms as unilateral blackouts in one eye
         b. Embolism–possible associations with rheumatic or arteriosclerotic heart disease, bacterial endocarditis, myocardial infarction, or septic focus in lungs
         c. Occlusion–middle cerebral occlusion affecting primarily the arm and face, anterior cerebral occlusion affecting primarily the leg
         d. Subdural hematoma–spontaneous or following trauma
      (2) Tumor–gradual onset of symptoms; lesions include intrinsic astrocytoma and glioblastoma, extrinsic meningioma, and lung metastasis
      (3) Diffuse demyelinative disease
         a. Schilder's type
         b. Pelizaeus-Merzbacher type
         c. Krabbe type
         d. Metachromatic leukoencephalopathy
         e. Progressive multifocal leukoencephalopathy
         f. Spongy degeneration of the brain
      (4) Migraine
   C. Occipital lesions–congruous field defect and macular sparing most likely

(1) Vascular lesions
  a. Occlusion of posterior cerebral artery–thrombotic or embolic
  b. Arteriovenous anomalies
  c. Aneurysms (rare)
  d. Subclavian steal syndrome, with reversal of blood flow through the vertebral artery
(2) Tumors–gradual onset of symptoms; lesions include intrinsic astrocytoma and glioblastoma, extrinsic meningioma, and lung metastasis
(3) Demyelinative disease
  a. Schilder's type
  b. Pelizaeus-Merzbacher type
  c. Krabbe type
  d. Metachromatic leukoencephalopathy
  e. Progressive multifocal leukoencephalopathy
  f. Spongy degeneration of the brain
(4) Trauma
  a. Direct–penetrating missiles and depressed bone fragments
  b. Indirect–general concussion syndrome
(5) Poisons such as carbon monoxide, digitalis, mescal, opium, lysergic acid diethylamide (LSD)
(6) Migraine

Cogan, D. G.: Neurology of the Visual System, 3rd ed. Springfield, Charles C Thomas, 1966, pp. 249, 256, 262, 290, 296.

Friedman, B.: Migraine: With Special Reference to Scintillating Scotoma. Eye Ear Nose Throat Monthly 50:52-58, 1971.

Harrington, D. O.: The Visual Fields, 3rd ed. St. Louis, C. V. Mosby, 1971.

Roy, F. H.: Ocular Differential Diagnosis, 2nd ed. Philadelphia, Lea & Febiger, 1975, pp. 510-512.

Smith, J. L.: Homonymous Hemianopsia. A Review of 100 Cases. Amer. J. Ophthal. 54:616, 1962.

Trobe, J. D., Lorber, M. L., and Schlezinfier, N. S.: Isolated Homonymous Hemianopia. Arch. Ophthal. 89:377-381, 1973.

ANATOMICAL LOCATION

Optic Tract Lesions—visual conduction system posterior to optic chiasm and anterior to lateral geniculate body, lesion demonstrating incongruous field defect on side opposite from defect often with decreased vision (80% accurate)

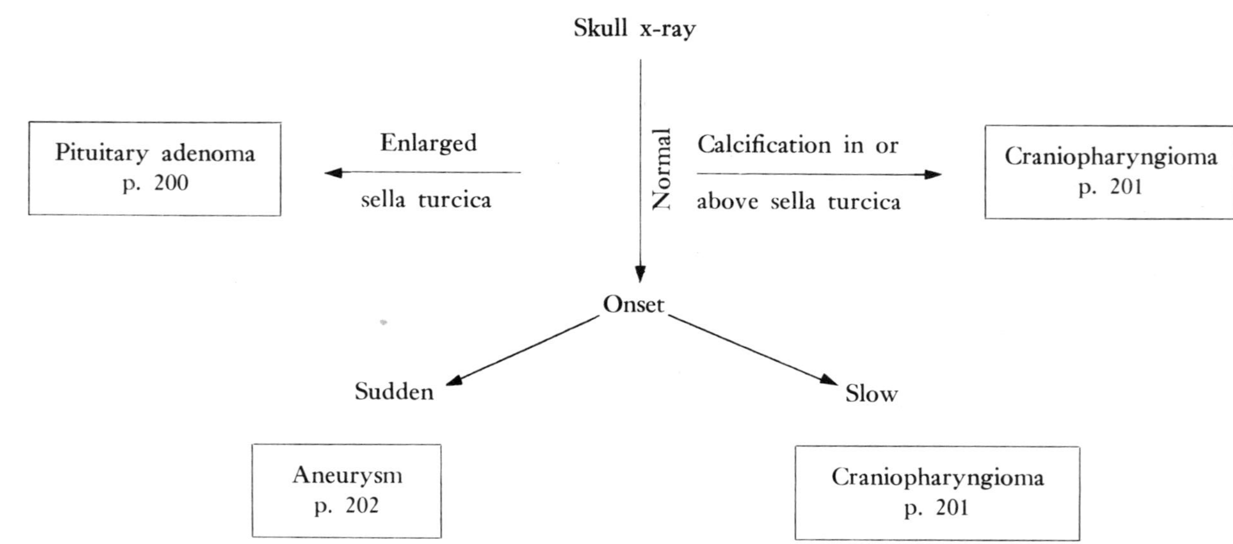

Temporal Lobe Lesions—homonymous field defect of side opposite from abnormality which frequently start in the upper quadrant. Clinical features include third nerve palsy, vertigo, confusion, loss of memory and dreamlike states. Excitatory lesions cause auras of odors and tastes (uncinate fits). Negative (symmetrical) optokinetic nystagmus (80% accurate)

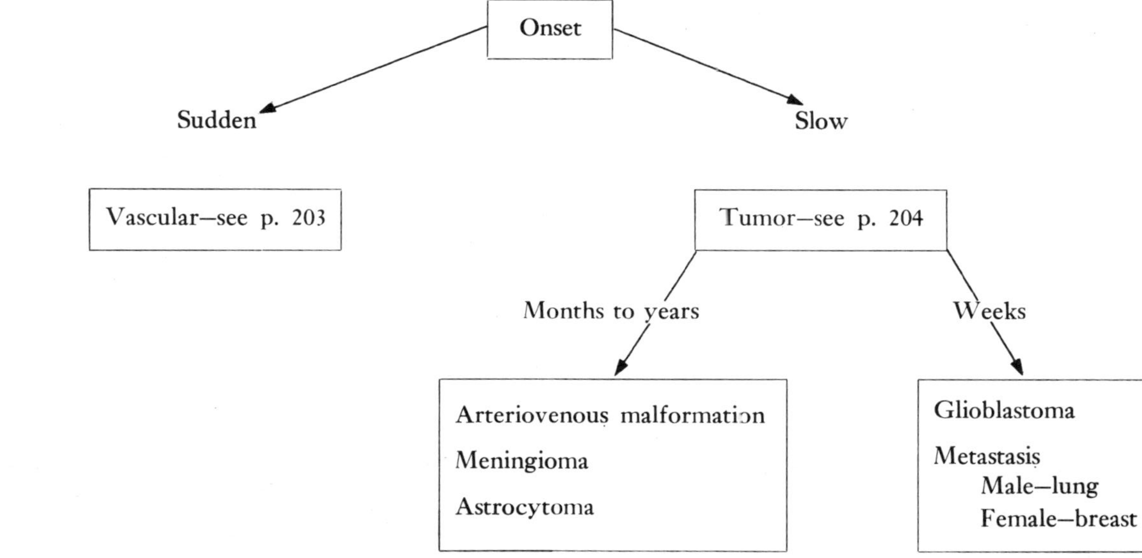

Parietal Lobe Lesions—homonymous field defect on side opposite from abnormality which begin in the lower visual quadrant. Positive (asymmetrical response) optokinetic nystagmus. Clinical picture includes deficient two-point discrimination, faulty tactile recognition of forms and shapes (astereognosis) and loss of position sense on side opposite to the lesion. If dominant hemisphere is involved, loss of visual work recognition, inability to write and inability to recognize whole words or symbols are noted (80% accurate)

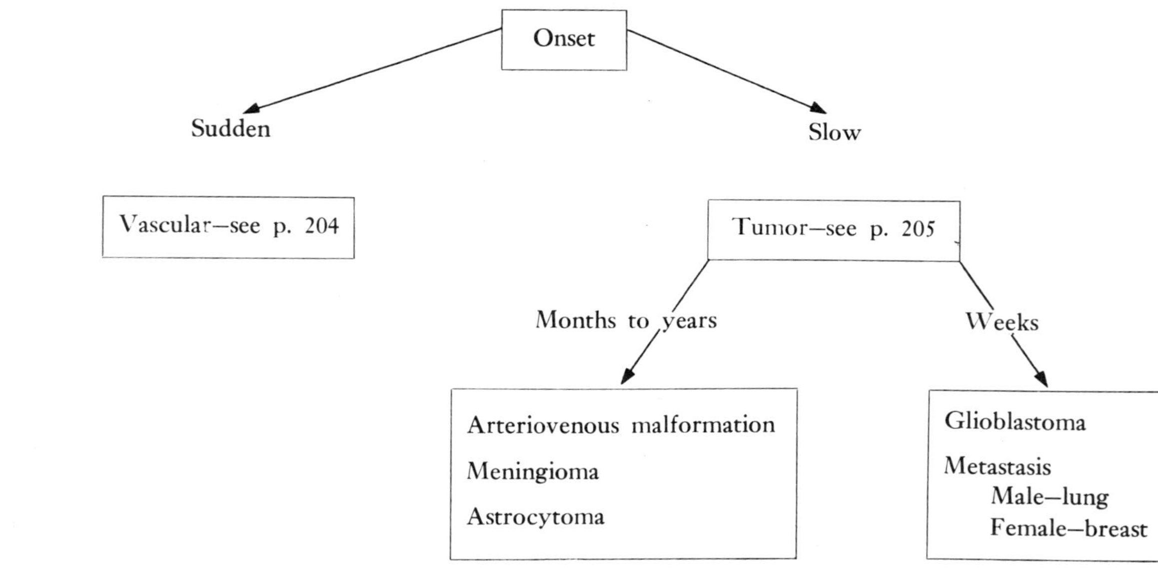

Occipital Lobe Lesions—congruous homonymous field defect side opposite from abnormality. Negative (symmetrical response) optokinetic nystagmus. Absent neurological signs or symptoms other than visual. Papilledema frequently present with tumor. Primitive hallucinations may be present (80% accurate)

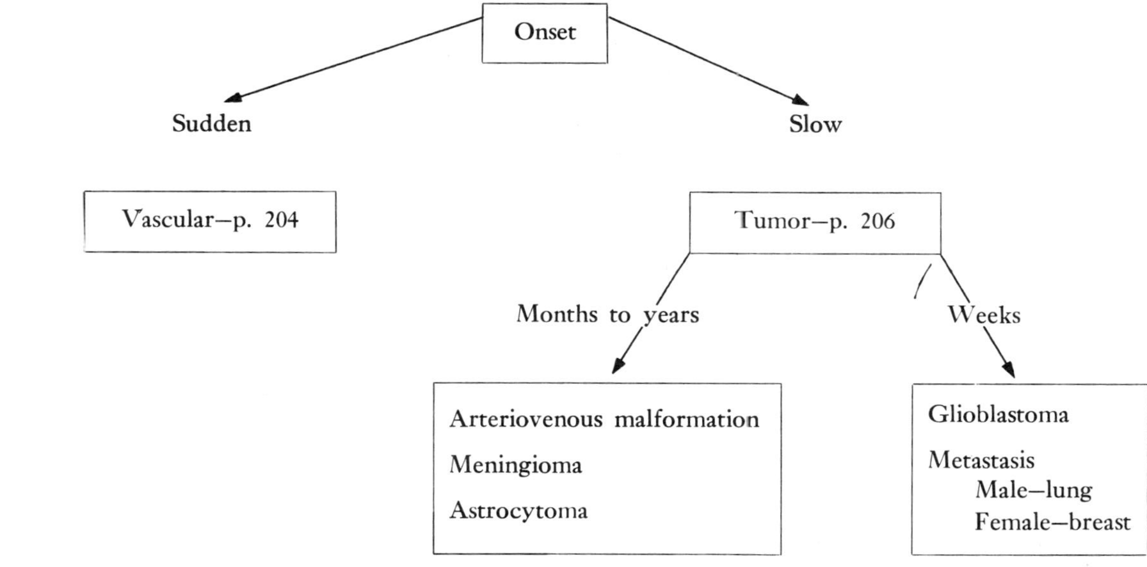

SPECIFIC DISORDERS

Pituitary Adenoma—usually benign tumor of pituitary gland

1. Clinical characteristics
   A. Visual fields
      (1) Bitemporal hemianopia–fairly symmetrical, and may have bitemporal central scotomas. Visual acuity may be normal or reduced (posterior chiasm)
      (2) Blindness in one eye and temporal hemianopia in other eye (more frequent above)–may have pallor of most affected optic nerve (anterior chiasm)
      (3) Homonymous hemianopia – reduced vision and/or atrophy of optic tract
   B. X-rays–enlarged sella turcica
   C. Endocrine dysfunction
      (1) Chromophobe adenoma–no endocrine symptoms or panhypopituitarism manifest by amenorrhea, impotence, loss of libido, fatigue or drowsiness
      (2) Acidiphilic adenomas–increased growth hormone production causing gigantism if in the first two decades. If later, acromegaly with prominence of jaw, thickness of tongue, enlargement of hands or feet, separation of teeth, coarseness of hair, deepening of voice, insulin-resistant diabetes mellitus and elevated serum phosphorus
      (3) Basophilic adenomas – hyperadrenalism (Cushing's disease) with moon facies, hypertension, acne, and insulin-resistant diabetes mellitus. Rarely, visual field defects or enlarged sella

2. Treatment–refer to neurologist or neurosurgeon
   A. Visual field and x-ray study
   B. Additional workup–arteriogram, pneumoencephalogram
   C. Surgery of pituitary through the frontal or transphenoidal approach (usually recommended with visual field defect)
   D. X-ray therapy–basophilic tumors more sensitive

Cogan, D. G.: Neurology of the Visual System. Springfield, Charles C Thomas, 1968, pp. 226-232.

Walsh, F. B. and Hoyt, W. F.: Clinical Neuro-Ophthalmology, 3rd ed., Vol. 3. Baltimore, Williams & Wilkins, 1969, pp. 2130-2154.

Huber, A.: Eye Symptoms in Brain Tumors, 2nd ed. St. Louis, C. V. Mosby, 1971, p. 189-211.

Craniopharyngioma—benign epithelial tumor or cyst derived from hypophyseal stalk

1. Clinical characteristics
   A. Visual fields
      (1) Bitemporal hemianopia
      (2) Blindness in one eye and temporal hemianopia in the other eye
      (3) Central or paracentral scotoma
      (4) Homonymous hemianopia of tract origin with reduced vision and/or optic atrophy
   B. Children—papilledema, vomiting, severe headache with increased intracranial pressure and hydrocephalus; hypopituitary signs of dwarfism, hypogenitalism or diabetes insipidus
   C. Adult—visual field changes (see above) or decrease in visual acuity; hypopituitarism (sexual disturbances, adiposity, soft skin, loss of axillary and pubic hair, and scanty growth of beard in males)
   D. "Characteristic lack of characteristics"—fluctuate widely
   E. X-rays—sella turcica may be enlarged; calcification in or above sella turcica highly suggestive, occurs more commonly in children than in adults

2. Treatment—refer to neurologist or neurosurgeon
   A. Additional workup—arteriogram, pneumoencephalogram
   B. Substitution therapy
      (1) Pitressin for diabetes
      (2) Steroids for adrenal insufficiency
      (3) Growth hormone for dwarfism
   C. Surgery if visual or other symptoms warrant it
   D. Treatment of hydrocephalus with shunt
   E. Radiation

Cogan, D. G.: Neurology of the Visual System. Springfield, Charles C Thomas, 1968, pp. 233-238.

Huber, A.: Eye Symptoms in Brain Tumors, 2nd ed. St. Louis, C. V. Mosby, 1971, pp. 211-218.

Walsh, F. B. and Hoyt, W. F.: Clinical Neuro-Ophthalmology, 3rd ed., Vol. 3. Baltimore, Williams & Wilkins, 1969, pp. 2157-2162.

Aneurysm of Internal Carotid

1. Clinical characteristics
   A. Intermittent, sudden and severe headache, supraorbital pain, and ophthalmoplegia (third, fourth and fifth nerve palsy)
   B. Acute onset, sudden deterioration as well as improvement of vision
   C. Visual fields
      (1) Blindness in one eye and temporal defect in other eye, defect more dense above than below; unilateral loss of vision and optic atrophy
      (2) Homonymous hemianopia with decreased vision and/or optic atrophy of tract origin
      (3) Nasal field defect
2. Arteriography—demonstrates aneurysm or bleeding areas (diagnostic)
3. Treatment—refer to neurologist or neurosurgeon
   A. Watch
   B. Clip artery

Cogan, D. G.: Neurology of the Visual System. Springfield, Charles C Thomas, 1968, p. 244.

Huber, A.: Eye Symptoms in Brain Tumors, 2nd ed. St. Louis, C. V. Mosby, 1971, pp. 297-299.

Walsh, F. B. and Hoyt, W. F.: Clinical Neuro-Ophthalmology, 3rd ed., Vol. 2. Baltimore, Williams & Wilkins, 1969, pp. 1778-1782.

Meningioma of Chiasm Region

1. Clinical characteristics
   A. Visual fields
      (1) Blindness in one eye and temporal hemianopia in other eye, pallor of most affected optic nerve and decreased or absent vision

(2) Bitemporal hemianopia

B. Proptosis with orbital invasion

C. Loss of smell on side of lesion

D. Headache

E. Slow progression

F. X-rays–hyperostosis or osteoporosis of tuberculum

2. Arteriography–helpful in that major vessels (carotid siphon and anterior cerebral artery) pushed upward and vessels in meningioma during venous phase show continued uptake of contrast media

3. Treatment–refer to neurologist or neurosurgeon

A. Early recognition

B. Surgical excision

Cogan, D. G.: Neurology of the Visual System. Springfield, Charles C Thomas, 1968, pp. 238-242.

Huber, A.: Eye Symptoms in Brain Tumors, 2nd ed. St. Louis, C. V. Mosby, 1971, pp. 218-225.

Walsh, F. B. and Hoyt, W. F.: Clinical Neuro-Ophthalmology, 3rd ed., Vol. 3. Baltimore, Williams & Wilkins, 1969, pp. 2262-2279.

Partial Carotid Occlusion—atherosclerosis most common cause

1. Clinical characteristics

A. Visual field changes–homonymous visual field defect on side opposite to lesion

B. Unilateral transient blindness (amaurosis fugax) lasting 2 to 10 minutes

C. Hemiplegia opposite to side of visual field involvement and on same side as lesion

D. Bruit over supraclavicular area on affected side, ipsilateral or contralateral side of neck

E. Cholesterol emboli in retinal blood vessels (Hollenhorst plaques)

F. Ophthalmodynamometry–retinal diastolic pressure 15% lower on affected side

G. Arteriography–determination of site of occlusion

2. Treatment—refer to neurologist or neurosurgeon
   A. Additional studies
   B. Hypertensive—normalizes blood pressure
   C. Anticoagulants—debatable
   D. Surgery to remove obstruction in selected cases

Cogan, D. G.: Neurology of the Visual System. Springfield, Charles C Thomas, 1968, pp. 37, 187, 280.

Walsh, F. B. and Hoyt, W. F.: Clinical Neuro-Ophthalmology, 3rd ed., Vol. 2. Baltimore, Williams & Wilkins, 1969, pp. 1802-1835.

Posterior Cerebral Artery Occlusion

1. Clinical characteristics
   A. Acute onset
   B. Total blindness at onset and within minutes homonymous hemianopia opposite from site of lesion
   C. Site of occlusion determined by arteriography
2. Treatment—refer to neurologist or neurosurgeon
   A. Additional studies
   B. Hypertensive—normalizes blood pressure
   C. Anticoagulants—debatable
   D. Surgery to remove obstruction in selected cases

Cogan, D. G.: Neurology of the Visual System. Springfield, Charles C Thomas, 1968, p. 281.

Walsh, F. B. and Hoyt, W. F.: Clinical Neuro-Ophthalmology, 3rd ed., Vol. 2. Baltimore, Williams & Wilkins, 1969, p. 1843.

Temporal Lobe Tumors—slow onset

1. Onset
   A. Weeks to months—glioblastoma or metastasis (males from lung and females from breast)
   B. Months to years—arteriovenous malformation, meningioma or astrocytoma
2. Clinical characteristics
   A. Visual field defect of homonymous hemianopia of side opposite from defect and frequently beginning in upper quadrant of visual fields

B. Headache frequent but rarely constant and usually widespread
C. Excitatory lesions causing auras of odors and tastes (uncinate fits)
D. Other clinical features–third nerve palsy, vertigo, confusion, loss of memory, dreamlike states, and highly differentiated formed hallucinations
E. Papilledema
F. Arteriography–major vessels deviated and vessels in tumor during venous phase show continued uptake of contrast media
G. Negative (symmetrical) optokinetic nystagmus

3. Treatment–refer to neurologist or neurosurgeon
   A. Additional tests as EEG and brain scan
   B. Early recognition
   C. Surgical excision
   D. X-ray therapy in selected cases
   E. Drugs as cyclophosphamide, mechlorethamine, methotrexate, prednisone and Atabrine

Cogan, D. G.: Neurology of the Visual System. Springfield, Charles C Thomas, 1968, pp. 282, 300.

Huber, A.: Eye Symptoms in Brain Tumors, 2nd ed. St. Louis, C. V. Mosby, 1971, pp. 166-175.

Walsh, F. B. and Hoyt, W. F.: Clinical Neuro-Ophthalmology, 3rd ed., Vol. 3. Baltimore, Williams & Wilkins, 1969, pp. 2175-2191, 2262-2279.

Parietal Lobe Tumors—slow onset

1. Onset
   A. Weeks to months–glioblastoma or metastasis (males from lung and females from breast)
   B. Months to years–arteriovenous malformation, meningioma or astrocytoma

2. Clinical characteristics
   A. Homonymous hemianopia of side opposite from defect which may begin in lower quadrant of visual field
   B. Positive (asymmetrical response) optokinetic nystagmus

C. Clinical disturbances–deficient two-point discrimination, faulty tactile recognition of forms and shapes of objects (astereognosis) and loss of position sense on side opposite to the lesion

D. If dominant hemisphere is involved, visual agnosia with loss of visual word recognition, inability to write, and inability to recognize whole words or symbols

E. Headache and papilledema

F. Arteriography–major vessels deviated and vessels in tumor during venous phase show continued uptake of contrast media

3. Treatment–refer to neurologist and neurosurgeon
   A. Additional tests as EEG and brain scan
   B. Early recognition
   C. Surgical excision
   D. X-ray therapy in selected cases
   E. Drugs as cyclophosphamide, mechlorethamine, methotrexate, prednisone and Atabrine

Cogan, D. G.: Neurology of the Visual System. Springfield, Charles C Thomas, 1968, pp. 282, 300.

Huber, A.: Eye Symptoms in Brain Tumors, 2nd ed. St. Louis, C. V. Mosby, 1971, pp. 175-179.

Walsh, F. B. and Hoyt, W. F.: Clinical Neuro-Ophthalmology, 3rd ed., Vol. 3. Baltimore, Williams & Wilkins, 1969, pp. 2191-2195, 2203-2206.

Occipital Lobe Tumors—slow onset

1. Onset
   A. Weeks to months–glioblastoma or metastasis (males from lung and females from breast)
   B. Months to years–arteriovenous malformation, meningioma or astrocytoma

2. Clinical characteristics
   A. Congruous field showing homonymous hemianopia on side opposite the defect
   B. Absent neurological symptoms other than visual, including unformed hallucinations
   C. Negative (symmetrical) optokinetic nystagmus

D. Headache and papilledema
E. Arteriography–major vessels deviated and vessels in tumor during venous phase show continued uptake of contrast media

3. Treatment–refer to neurologist or neurosurgeon
   A. Additional test as EEG, lumbar puncture
   B. Early recognition
   C. Surgical excision
   D. X-ray therapy in selected cases
   E. Drugs as cyclophosphamide, mechlorethamine, methotrexate, prednisone and Atabrine

Cogan, D. B.: Neurology of the Visual System. Springfield, Charles C Thomas, 1968, pp. 282, 300.

Huber, A.: Eye Symptoms in Brain Tumors, 2nd ed. St. Louis, C. V. Mosby, 1971, pp. 179-186.

Walsh, F. B. and Hoyt, W. F.: Clinical Neuro-Ophthalmology, 3rd ed., Vol. 3. Baltimore, Williams & Wilkins, 1969, pp. 2195-2203.

Index